KU-020-739

2|23

It's All in the Head

It's All in the Head

Majella O'Donnell

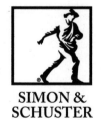

**SIMON &
SCHUSTER**

London · New York · Sydney · Toronto · New Delhi

A CBS COMPANY

First published in Great Britain by Simon & Schuster UK Ltd, 2014
A CBS COMPANY

Copyright © 2014 by Majella O'Donnell

This book is copyright under the Berne Convention.
No reproduction without permission.
All rights reserved.

The right of Majella O'Donnell to be identified as the author
of this work has been asserted by her in accordance with sections
77 and 78 of the Copyright, Designs and Patents Act, 1988.

5 7 9 10 8 6 4

Simon & Schuster UK Ltd
1st Floor
222 Gray's Inn Road
London WC1X 8HB

www.simonandschuster.co.uk

Simon & Schuster Australia, Sydney
Simon & Schuster India, New Delhi

A CIP catalogue record for this book
is available from the British Library

Hardback ISBN: 978-1-4711-3933-8
Trade paperback ISBN: 978-1-4711-3894-2
eBook ISBN: 978-1-4711-3896-6

The author and publishers have made all reasonable efforts to
contact copyright-holders for permission, and apologise for
any omissions or errors in the form of credits given.
Corrections may be made to future printings.

Typeset by M Rules
Printed and bound by CPI Group (UK) Ltd, Croydon, CR0 4YY

To my children, Siobhán and Michael:

I hope the journey wasn't too bumpy

To the first person I ever loved, my mother:

thank you

To my husband, Daniel:

what can I say that you don't already know

To my Dad:

I miss you

CONTENTS

PREFACE

When it was suggested to me that I write a book, at first I thought to myself, what could I possibly have to say that would be of interest to anyone else? I always thought that books were written by highly intellectual people, who have great imaginations and verbal skills and lots of patience – and I certainly wouldn't put myself into that category! But then I thought about it and realized that ever since I had spoken openly about my experience with depression and my journey with breast cancer, a huge number of people had contacted me to say that my openness had been very helpful to them. The word 'inspirational' was the one most people used. Imagine. *Me*. Inspirational. An ordinary girl from a small town in Tipperary with a very normal upbringing. I began to think that maybe my writing a book wasn't such a crazy idea after all.

I've had a lot of ups and downs, as all of us have. There's nothing special about that. What I aim to do in this book is to tell you how it was for me and what I did to make changes in my life to stop becoming a 'poor-me' kind of person and to take responsibility for my own circumstances. I do not by any means claim to be an expert on depression or anxiety or any other mental health issues or for that matter, cancer and all that goes with it, but what I can talk about is my experience with both and how I dealt with, and am still dealing with, mind and body.

I have given some talks on my experience with depression and people have always said that they can identify with me. I must have a way of explaining things that people can connect with. I have enjoyed what I have done so far and I feel that maybe that's my calling in life. It is a huge responsibility and I do notice that people approach me with their problems in the hope that I can tell them what to do to fix things but, unfortunately, I can't. I wish I could. All I can do is share what I have experienced and what I did to help myself and if other people can use that information to help themselves, that's wonderful.

When I set out to write this book, I wanted to look at

the milestones in my life and how they've shaped me and made me who I am: the good and the bad, the struggles and the successes. For me, that's what it's all about: not the destination, but the journey and the milestones along the way. If, by writing this book, I can help others on their journey through life, I'll be a happy woman.

[signature] xo

Chapter 1

MY HEAD SHAVE AND
THE LATE LATE SHOW

'You've done it! You've absolutely done it!' Ryan Tubridy said, holding my hand. I was so glad to hear those words because I knew then that it was over. My hair had all been shaved off. I had done what I set out to do and now I was sitting in front of hundreds of thousands of people, absolutely bald. I know that I should probably have felt elated, or upset at the loss of my hair, but instead, all I felt was relief. I'd set myself the task of having my head shaved on live television, and now, I'd actually gone through with it. It felt like such a milestone.

It was 14 September 2013, and I had been diagnosed with breast cancer on 12 July that year. I will talk about my cancer journey in more detail later on in the book, but because of the impact that my appearance that night on *The Late Late Show* had and because so many people responded in such a positive way, I feel that I should explain why I did the head shave.

Following my diagnosis, I had had lumpectomy surgery at the end of July 2013. My oncologist then advised that, having had some tests done, I should have a course of chemotherapy to minimize the possibility of the cancer returning. At the time, I was very surprised that I needed chemo. I suppose I thought that it was a bit extreme. I had found my lump at an early stage and I thought that would mean I wouldn't need it. I understood that chemo was only administered if your cancer had progressed, but I was going to take all the advice and help I could get because, after all, they were the experts.

I was lying in bed about a week before the first course of treatment was due to start, in September, feeling a little apprehensive because I'd heard how ill chemo could make you feel and I wondered how I'd react. My husband, Daniel, had left to do a tour in America at the end of August, so I was on my own, with no distractions – usually the two of us catch up on the day's events and chat away at that time in the evening. I started to slip into that pre-sleep phase, when you're not quite asleep, but not fully awake either and you have lucid dreams. All of a sudden, I was wide awake, with a very clear idea in my head. It was as quick as that and certainly not premeditated. The thought was that I should shave my hair on live television to raise money for charity and to raise awareness of breast cancer. I didn't know where the idea had come from and at first, I almost dismissed it. I can be very spontaneous at times and sometimes it's not a good thing! I thought that maybe I was being ridiculous and that no one would want to be involved with something as personal as that on live television, but I'm a fairly brazen woman and I'll usually try anything that's thrown at me. I believe that life is for living and the more we can experience in life, the better. I want to leave this world feeling that I have accomplished something worthwhile and I believe that sometimes you have to take risks to achieve that. So, I went to sleep with the idea firmly set in my mind. I was going to give it a go.

When I woke up the next morning, I was almost frantic about getting the head shave organized. I knew that I had very little time, so I had to contact people straight away. I knew that I would not be in great form once chemo started and that my hair would start to fall out anyway and I really didn't want that to happen. I wanted to call Daniel to see what his reaction would be, but he was about eight hours behind in the States, so I called a businessman friend of mine and told him what I had planned and asked if he knew of any companies that would be interested in sponsoring me.

'What kind of money are you hoping to raise?' he asked. I told him that around the €10,000 mark would be great.

'Hmm …' he said. 'That's quite a modest amount.' I think he was very cautious about the idea, but then again, who wouldn't be? He must have thought I was a bit crazy to even think of doing such a thing. He was probably also a little worried that I was going to do something that I might regret. 'Leave it with me and I'll get back to you,' he said diplomatically. I suppose I thought that maybe one company would come on board and that they could get publicity of some sort in return for sponsoring me.

Once that call was made, I felt absolutely sure that I was doing the right thing and I was really hoping that Daniel would agree. I don't have to 'ask permission' from Daniel to do anything, but I always want and respect his opinion and he always gives good advice.

My next call was to *The Late Late Show* researcher John Downes, whom I knew from having appeared on the show previously. I knew that by appearing on the biggest talk/entertainment show in the country, I would reach the largest audience and have the best chance of raising as much money as possible for charity. I also thought that as it was a very radical thing to do, they would certainly consider it. I explained what I had in mind and John said he would get back to me later on that day. I think he was pleased that I had called because my diagnosis had been reported in the papers, but I had not spoken personally to anyone about it up to that point. *The Late Late Show* would be glad of the opportunity to interview me exclusively, I thought, and I had a good relationship with them, which also helped.

John called me back later and said that they would do an interview: they thought people would be interested to know how I was dealing with the diagnosis. I corrected him and said that I wanted to do a head shave, *not* an interview. I was really adamant that this was *not* about me personally, but that I was just someone with a voice, who could do some good. He was fairly surprised as he hadn't realized that I wanted to actually *do* the head shave, not just talk about it! I explained that it had to be done as soon as possible because I was starting the chemo the following week. John promised to go away and talk about this with the *Late Late* team and that he would come back to me the next day. I think at that stage he was excited, but also unsure if it would work, as something like that had never been done before.

That evening, Daniel called and I told him about my idea. As I said earlier, I sometimes come up with fairly wacky ideas and Daniel usually smiles and says something like, 'Do ya know what? You're something else.' This was no exception. I explained the thoughts behind my head shave. I told him that the idea really wasn't a conscious one, but one I felt I was drawn to and that it would be a great way to make something positive out of losing my hair, which is a pretty negative thing. He thought it was a great idea, but told me I was aiming far too low with the target I had in mind. If I was willing to go on live television and do that, with my profile, then I should be looking at raising €100,000, he suggested.

I thought he was mad. 'People don't have a lot of spare cash these days, Daniel. It would be very hard to raise that amount, but I'll compromise and raise the target to fifty thousand euro.'

'Are you sure you want to go ahead and do this?' he asked. When I said yes, he said, 'What if people are upset by it and it gets a bad reaction?' I told him that I was doing it for all the right reasons and that if it did get a bad reaction, I would deal with it then. I knew that it might offend some people, but I felt strongly that the majority would support and get what I was doing. I also felt that the signal or idea to do the head shave had come from a higher being, so I felt I was in safe hands. I am not a hugely religious person, but I do believe that there is a God and that gives me great strength in good and bad times. I believe that I was guided to do this because of the good it would do for other people.

The next day, John called back and said that they would be willing to do the head shave, but he insisted on an interview as well. He also told me that I would have to make it clear that it was my idea and that I had not been pressurized into it. I thought, how on earth could anyone think I could be pressurized into something like that! I assured him that I would make that very clear. We then talked about the content of the interview because, as I said, I did not want it to be about me, but about all the people out there who had to go through the same thing every day all around Ireland. Unfortunately, cancer is a very common illness these days: one in three Irish people will get cancer at one stage during their lifetime, according to the Irish Cancer Society. I wanted people to see that it was OK, and that the hair loss that comes with some types of chemo is also OK; it doesn't have to be a devastating experience. We can either think of shaving our heads as the worst possible thing in the world, or we can choose to believe that it is just something that has to be done. I made the choice to get on with it. I knew my hair was going to grow back again in six months' time, so for me, it wasn't that big a deal. People who suffer from alopecia can lose their hair and never get it back. That, to me, would be a far more traumatic thing to deal with. I was the lucky one as far as my hair was concerned.

John then explained that it would be very important to do the interview first so that the whole thing could be put into context. I agreed, and I'm so glad I did: a lot of people have said that it was the interview that struck a chord with them, followed by the head shave, because it gave them a greater understanding of why I was doing it. Maybe just doing the head shave on its own would have been too stark. I didn't agree with his suggestion that we do the interview in the first segment of the show and come back later on to do the shave, though: I knew that if I had time between the interview and the shave, I would think about what I was doing and that would be a disaster. I could fall to pieces if I really thought about it. No, I had to plough straight into it, I knew, with no time allowed for what was happening to really sink in.

I must say that everyone working on *The Late Late Show* was absolutely wonderful and very respectful at all times.

Because I was having the chemotherapy the day before the show, I wasn't sure how I would feel, but I had been told that because of the steroids I would be taking, I should be fine on the Friday as the full effects of the treatment wouldn't yet have kicked in. So it was decided that I would be interviewed at the end of the first segment, get set up for the shave during the first break, and then come back after the break and go straight into it.

Now that I knew that *The Late Late Show* was on board, I needed to contact someone at the Irish Cancer Society. John had asked if I had a charity in mind and I knew I wanted the funds raised to go to The Irish Cancer Society because I understood that their previous national fund raising day had been a complete washout, due to poor weather, and they were down by about €700,000 on their target: they really needed a boost. Daniel had previously been involved with the Donegal Relay for Life event, a twenty-four-hour walking relay, which is held every year in the county to raise funds for the Irish Cancer Society and he had met CEO John McCormack. When I called John to introduce myself and to tell him my plans, he was absolutely delighted. We decided to meet, along with John Downes from *The Late Late Show*, Mark Mellett, Head of Fundraising and Kathleen O'Meara, Head of Advocacy and Communications at the

Irish Cancer Society. I knew that if we were to make the most of this opportunity, we had to be well organized. I keep saying 'we' when I should, in fact, say 'they', because other than arriving at the studios and shaving my head, all the other hard work had to be delegated to these people.

We met on a Monday and the show was on the following Friday. By Wednesday, they had an area on their website with my picture on it, where people could donate just to that specific event and they already had a phone number to which people could text their donation. 'Text "Pink" to 50300'. I will never forget that number! If it had not been so straightforward, the money raised would have been far less. Remember that at this stage, we had no idea whatsoever what the reaction would be like. We didn't know if two hundred and fifty people would call or two thousand five hundred! It's very hard to gauge something like that when you have no previous model to work on. However, I left the meeting that day even more convinced that this was what I should be doing.

Up to this point, I hadn't sat down and fully thought through what I would be doing. I suppose I was more concerned about the chemotherapy session that was taking place on the Thursday before the show. I had no idea what to expect, but, like the head shave, I tried not to think about it. If you think too much about what you imagine things will be like, you can really get yourself into a state, which is pointless. Our imaginations are usually a lot worse than reality. My motto is to wait until I am in the situation, whatever it is, and then deal with the reality of it.

I had to take steroids for three days around the chemo: the day before, the day of and the day after. They can make you feel pretty invincible, so when the Thursday arrived and I went in for my first chemotherapy session, I felt grand. I am a very curious person, so I love finding out the whys and hows and wheres of everything, so I was interested in how the whole chemo process worked. A lot of people don't want to know the nitty-gritty, but I'm the opposite. I want to know how things work, what the effects are and what their purpose is, then I always feel in a better position to make choices.

As Daniel was away on tour, my mother came with me for my first chemotherapy session at the Beacon Hospital, where I was being treated. I was there about ten minutes when Kathleen, Daniel's sister, suddenly arrived into the room. I was really pleased to see her and amazed that she had driven down from Donegal just to be there with me on my first day. She has been a wonderful support throughout the whole cancer journey.

I was surprised by how normal everyone in the chemo area looked and how normally they behaved. They were just sitting reading their papers or talking to friends or family members. Nobody was in obvious pain or distress, as I had been expecting. Of course, now I know that if you are in any way sick, you won't be able to have your chemo, so everyone is in relatively good form at these sessions.

I found a seat in a corner and I sat there until the nurse came over and asked me if I wanted to order breakfast or lunch, which pleased me because I knew that they didn't expect me to be sick. I started to feel more and more relaxed all the time. The nurses are so friendly and encouraging and they really help you to feel safe. I am also very lucky because I have no problem with needles at all. I listened to everything they said and once the cannula was in, I was fine. You need the loo a lot because of all the fluids they put into you, but you can walk around with the drip or disconnect it if you need to. The chemotherapy took about three hours and it really didn't take much out of me at all. To my surprise, I was even able to go to Dundrum Shopping Centre afterwards to find something to wear for the big night.

That was another decision that I had to give some thought to. I didn't want to look too dolled-up, as if I was going on a night out. That was not the image I wanted to portray. This was a serious statement and a fundraiser and I knew I needed to convey that. I also didn't want to look like a frump! I know I'm not the most glamorous of people, but I wanted to look reasonably 'up to date' as they say, but I didn't want to show cleavage or legs and I wanted to look respectful under the circumstances. I chose a dress that had long sleeves with a high neck and I wore it with black tights. That would do fine.

Next was my make-up.

I imagined myself without hair and I knew that my face and eyes would then be the focus of attention. I have always had big eyes, which I hated when I was young, but as I have got older, I have learned to love them. I wanted them to 'pop out' to distract from the lack of hair, so I enlisted the help of a make-up artist called Zoë Clark because I wanted a really professional look. Normally, I am pretty good at doing my own make-up, because shortly after I married Daniel, I went on a make-up course for a week to give me an idea of how to 'do' my face myself. I realized that we would be attending lots of different events and I didn't really have a clue how to do my make-up. It was one of the best things I ever did. I'm still not great, but I'm much better and I always do my own make-up now. However, this was a special event! I wanted someone who I knew could make me look as good as possible. And Zoë did. I have put a few pictures in the book and if you look at the one on the evening of the head shave, I look pretty good, if I say so myself. Trust me, I don't come any better than that!

Next was my hair.

Because I knew that it was all going to fall out, even before I decided to shave my head, I'd had it cut very short. I wanted to get used to looking at myself with very short hair and to take control of it. I have a good friend called John Maher, whom I have known for about twenty-three years. He has his own salon in Dublin called Queen Beauty Emporium and we get on really well. We have a very similar sense of humour and he is a very kind person. I wanted someone that I was very comfortable with to be with me on the set that night and I knew John was the very person. I called him and told him what I was doing and he said he would be proud to be part of it. (I'm sure he thought I was a little mad, too, but he never said!)

I wasn't sure what I wanted to do about my lack of hair. Because I didn't know what I would look like without my hair, it was hard to decide. Would I wear a wig or a scarf or hat? I liked the idea of wearing a wig, but one that was totally different to my usual hairstyle. I figured that, as I was losing my hair, I may as well go for it and enjoy having the kind of hair I'd always wanted. I went to a few places and tried on these beautiful long blonde curly wigs and then straight ones and dark ones and all sorts, but nothing seemed to suit me. I had always fancied having long flowing thick hair because my own hair is very fine, but every time I put on a wig like that, I looked ridiculous!! And I *mean* ridiculous. It really didn't suit my face at all. So, in the end, I gave in and thought I had better get something that was similar to my own hairstyle. I chose a short blonde bob, which was styled and ready to go on the night.

So that was it. I was all sorted, with dress, hair, wig and make-up.

When *The Late Late Show* asked me how many tickets I wanted for the show that night, I had another decision to make. I knew that if I was looking at my family while my head was being shaved, I would get very upset for myself and for them and I probably would break down in tears and not be able to control myself. I really didn't want that to happen. I also wanted their support when I came off the set and if they were in the audience, they would not be able to leave until the show was over. So it was decided that my mother, Marion, my sister, Jo, Daniel's sister, Kathleen, and my very good friend, Martina, would all watch the show on television in the green room. My son, Michael, was working in London at the time and I didn't want him to have to take time off to travel over to Dublin. My daughter, Siobhán, and my niece, Jane, were in Tenerife on holidays and staying with my dad. I was glad they weren't with me because I'm sure the night would have been very difficult for them and I didn't want that. I didn't want it for them or for me. I had enough to concentrate on without worrying about how they would react. I knew Jo could look after Mum, but Michael and Siobhán were different. They were my children and I knew they'd be terribly upset for me. I worried that the fact that I had cancer might not yet have sunk in with them and I was afraid that they might react badly because it would now be all too obvious that I had the disease. Up to that point, I still looked the same and I wasn't sick, but that was about to change in a very short space of time. When you see a bald woman, you always assume that she has cancer. There is no avoiding it. If they had been at the studio I would have had to concentrate on them and how they were reacting and I just didn't know if I would be able to do that. I mean, I wasn't even sure how *I* would react! I had to look after myself first on this occasion.

Friday arrived and I still felt fine after the chemotherapy.

I had been concerned that I would start to feel awful and that I wouldn't be able to do the show, but I would have needed to be really unwell to pull out. A car picked us up from our apartment about two hours before the show. I was very giddy and anxious and I just wanted to get to the studio as quickly as possible and get it all over with. It wasn't that I was dreading it: I was just over-excited and uncertain of the reaction and I wanted it to be over. I had organized for Zoë to meet me there and do the make-up just before the show: I wanted it to be as fresh as possible. The others went and got themselves a glass of wine and Zoë started the transformation.

Ryan Tubridy, who was hosting *The Late Late Show*, came to my dressing room and welcomed me and said that he thought what I was doing was extremely brave. He also told me that, if at any time I wanted to stop what was happening, I could do so. He was very nice, professional, and friendly and it made me feel very relaxed. I had no intention of stopping it, but the offer was there and I appreciated that.

As the time went on and the moment of the shave drew nearer, my mouth started to get very dry. I always get a dry mouth when I'm nervous. I couldn't drink any alcohol because of the treatment and normally that would be the first thing that I would have: a nice big glass of wine to help settle the nerves! I kept drinking water, but it didn't seem to help – the nerves were still very much there. I was wired up with a microphone and shortly afterwards the floor manager came to take me on set. I checked on my mum and friends and they were fine, eating canapés and drinking wine, but they were all nervous for me and Kathleen was a bit upset at the thought of what was happening. She is a very emotional person and wears her heart on her sleeve so she just got up and walked outside to gather herself. She knew that I couldn't cope with anyone else's emotions at that time.

I knew that the interview was coming first and that was not a problem. I don't feel nervous being interviewed on television because I don't think about all the people who might be watching. I just think of it as a conversation with the person that's interviewing me. I don't think about the cameras or anything like that. I never want to know what questions I'll be asked as I think its more natural if you answer instinctively and from the heart. Any time I have appeared on television, my biggest concern has been not to trip on the way to my seat. I always wonder what I would do if I fell on the way out. How embarrassing would that be?! And most of the time the floors in those studios are painted and highly polished, so you really do have to be careful as you walk out. I've done any number of interviews at this stage, but never quite get over that fear.

The moment had arrived at last. I was announced on and Ryan came out to welcome me. We sat and he asked me various questions about my cancer: how I had found the lump, how I was told about the cancer, how I reacted and how Daniel reacted upon hearing it. All the questions that I expected to be asked and I answered them to the best of my ability. I am always conscious that my experience may be very different to someone else's and I always want to make it very clear that I am only speaking on my own behalf and that I am no expert. Every cancer is different and every cancer patient reacts differently to the disease and the treatment.

The interview ended and we came to the break. The reality of what I was about to do had well and truly sunk in, and now I just had to wait.

My friend John came onto the set and they set up a table with the shaver on it and a chair for me to sit on. Ryan kept asking if I was OK and I was – I felt fine. Then John put a white hairdressing gown on me to cover my clothes and it suddenly hit me: Oh, my God, this is it! I thought. I started to lose control of things. The tears started to well up in my eyes, I had a lump in my throat and I began to shake. What on earth was I doing? I thought. I was about to have my head shaved in front of thousands of people. I thought of my family up in the green room, watching, of my father, Tom, and Siobhán, watching television in Tenerife and Michael, watching in London. Was I making a big mistake? Well, it was too late now to do anything about it. I got a tissue from John and dabbed my eyes and then Zoë, the make-up artist, came over and reminded me that the make-up would start to smudge if I was crying too much: that helped me to take control once more. Ryan asked again if I was OK and reminded me that if I didn't want to go ahead with it, they could always play some music instead. I said, 'No, I'm fine. Let's just do this'. The waiting was almost over, and the waiting is the worst part.

The second half of the show began and I sat in the chair and just concentrated on not crying. I kept telling myself that it would be fine and that I would be fine. Ryan asked John a couple of questions and then John started to shave. The noise of the shaver was another confirmation that it was definitely happening and then I started to see little bits of hair flying around my head and I understood that it was too late to back out now. As if he'd read my mind, Ryan asked me why I hadn't taken the opportunity to pull out, but I told him that once I decide on something, I like to see it through. I knew in my heart and soul that I would be glad in the end.

As John shaved, the phone and text numbers for donations were shown on screen. I still didn't know what sort of reaction I was getting – the audience was silent. When my hair was almost all gone, Ryan said, 'You look amazing, you really look amazing. You should see yourself.'

I asked the audience for reassurance: 'What do I look like?' The audience was fantastic and in response, they all started clapping. Then one man at the back of the audience stood up and quickly sat down again, but someone else saw him and stood up, too, and the next thing I saw was the whole audience on its feet. I couldn't believe the response. I didn't think that people would be that affected by what I had done and I couldn't help but feel emotional again.

Once the applause had died down, Ryan asked if I wanted to see myself, but I really didn't want to at this stage because I thought that I would look dreadful and that would knock whatever little confidence I had. I could look at myself later when nobody else was there and take a moment to come to terms with the new me. And as it would all be over at that stage, there would be nothing I could do about it. Then Ryan asked if I wanted to feel my head and it was the strangest, most liberating thing ever. It felt like velvet and it was strange to feel my skull right under my fingertips. I loved the feeling, I have to say. Someone in the audience shouted, 'Sinéad O'Connor, eat your heart out,' because I looked like Sinéad when she was bald, which made me laugh. My confidence was growing all the time. Ryan kept saying I looked great, so then I started to think that maybe I wouldn't need the wig after all. I'd brought it with me to put on after I'd had my head shaved, but I wondered if, after seeing me bald and liking it, the audience would think the wig was awful. In fact, most people did think I looked better without it, but I decided it didn't matter because I could always take the wig off whenever I liked.

When I was finished and left the set, people were congratulating me everywhere. I had some photos taken by the Irish Cancer Society and then I went to the green room to see how my mum was. She was very emotional and said she was very proud of me. I then called my father in Tenerife and his exact words were, 'You were bloody great!' I spoke to Siobhán and Michael and they were both fine: Siobhán was emotional, but she, too, said she was very proud to have me as her mum. I felt as if I was on cloud nine.

When I got a quiet moment, I went back down to the

dressing room and took the wig off to have my first look. It was fine and I was quite impressed really. I liked what I saw. I felt like a bit of a rebel. Like I was making a statement, which I suppose I was. 'Look at me. I have no hair and I don't care.' I thought that I had a nicely shaped head and that my ears didn't stick out. My new 'haircut' also showed my jawline and the shape of my face in a good light. I remember saying to myself: 'Thanks, Mum for a well-shaped head'! I don't think I will ever let my hair grow to any significant length again. It has grown a little now, but it's still very short. It seems to flatter me and it certainly takes a lot less time getting ready to go out. I would recommend short hair to every woman!

Later, I was told that the response was so fantastic that Irish Cancer Society website had crashed and that a lot of people had had trouble getting through. How amazing was that? People were just fantastic. They kept texting and calling and never gave up. Apparently, I was even trending on Twitter! The response far outweighed my expectations. Daniel was obviously right when he said I'd been aiming too low.

As soon as we were finished, we all went home, as I was feeling really tired and fairly drained after all that emotion. I slept well that night, but had to get up at one stage to put a little cap on as my head was really cold. I got used to that after a few days.

The next morning I had loads of texts and messages on Facebook telling me that what I had done was fantastic and how inspiring it was. There were thousands of comments and all of them were positive. That's pretty unusual, as there are always people that have a different view or negative people that have to put you down. It was quite refreshing. For some reason or other, most people will focus on the bad stuff and ignore the good and I'm no different. If I get one thousand positive comments and one negative comment, the negative one is the one that gets to me. That is something that I am still trying to 'let go of'.

The high of the *Late Late* lasted for another couple of days, but then the effects of the chemo took hold. It's really hard to describe exactly what the chemo did to me even to this day. It's like your brain can't function or gather any thoughts and to put words together takes real effort. I couldn't concentrate on anything and all I wanted to do was to lie down. On Monday morning, Ryan Tubridy's radio programme on RTÉ 2FM called to see if I would come on air to talk about the response to the *Late Late*. The thought of trying to have a conversation with Ryan felt too much because I could hardly speak. I just felt incapable of functioning, but I really wanted to go on and thank everyone for their kind donations and for their wonderful support. At this stage I had no idea how much money had been raised, but I was really hoping for the €50,000 mark.

On air, Ryan asked how I was and then said that €250,000 was a fantastic amount of money to raise. I thought that I had misheard him, so I asked again how much it was. When he said it again, I was genuinely absolutely shocked. I couldn't believe it. I started to feel a lump in my throat, the tears started and my voice went all wobbly. Even though I was beginning to feel really bad with the chemotherapy, I was elated. Now I knew for certain that what I had done was worthwhile and had been well received.

As the week went on and I began to feel worse and worse physically, the money being raised was increasing all the time. Newspaper, radio and television people all started to call and ask if I would do interviews, but I just couldn't and anyway, after my appearance on the *Late Late*, I just wanted to keep my head down and get on with the treatment. Even if I had wanted to be interviewed, I wouldn't have been able for it. By the end of the first week, €450,000 had been raised. I was truly astonished and delighted and it made that little thought that had jumped into my head the previous week and everything that had happened since seem worthwhile.

As I recovered from the first cycle of chemotherapy and started to go out again, people came up to me and congratulaed me on what I had done. They were always really kind and it's a lovely thing to be acknowledged in person. It makes you feel very humble. I truly believe that what I did was an easy thing. People kept telling me I was very brave and that I was an inspiration, but I didn't feel like that at all. I only had my head shaved, I kept insisting.

I was very lucky because my cancer was at an early stage and I have a great chance of making a full recovery. It is because of people donating money to cancer research that my chances of recovery have increased so significantly and I wanted to do my bit in the battle to conquer cancer. I have no doubt whatsoever that there are lots of people out there who would have jumped at the chance to do what I did had they the opportunity, but I know that I am in the public eye and that I have some sort of a voice, even if it's only a little one. I believe that it is my duty to use that voice to help other people in whatever way I can, if I can. I was privileged to be able to do so little and to help raise so much to help in the fight against cancer.

*

A week after *The Late Late Show* I received a beautiful bouquet of flowers with a card that read: 'This day last week you did something truly extraordinary, which we will never forget. Warm wishes for a speedy recovery from Ryan and all of *The Late Late Show* team'. I thought that was so thoughtful and sincere. Most TV stations would just be delighted that they got such a good response to their show, but think no further than that. To me, it showed real sincerity and that they actually did appreciate what I had done.

Ever since the head shave, people recognize me as myself rather than as Daniel's wife. I have received so many letters since I shaved my head and I am so grateful to everyone that took the time to send them. I have a very privileged life and it is amazing to think that so many people are aware of me and interested in my welfare when I don't even know them. It's probably easy to recognize me when I am walking around with a bald head!

The head shave has opened many avenues for me, including being given the opportunity to write this book, so I will never regret that I did it. I only wish I could do something like that every year, but it was a one-off event. Even if I got cancer again, I could never do that and have a similar reaction from people.

In November, I was nominated for the *Irish Tatler* magazine 'Woman of the Year' Awards under the 'Special Achievement' category. I had never won an award in my life before that, so it was a great honour.

Friday 13 September 2013 will always be a special day for me. It changed my life for the better and I will never forget it.

Chapter 2

CHILDHOOD

That Friday in September 2013 was a turning point in my life, a life which began fifty-three years earlier, in Thurles Town in Co. Tipperary. I was born on 14 April 1960 and my mother said I arrived at about three o'clock in the afternoon, while the sun was shining through the bedroom window. I was Thomas and Marion's third child and after two difficult births, Mum tells me that I arrived with little or no trouble. I'd like to say that I continued to be little or no trouble throughout my life, but that would be a lie!

From the word go, I was a live wire. I talked for Ireland (nothing has changed there then) and was always willing to entertain people in whatever way I could. I wanted to be involved in everything and I wanted to be liked by everyone. I have a brother four years older than me, Michael, and a sister two years older than me, Josephine or Jo. When I was ten years old we moved to Galway and my mother announced that she was expecting another baby. I remember being very excited, but also thinking how old she was, even though she was only thirty-three. In July 1970, my baby sister, Moira, was born and the family was complete. I treated her like a doll and loved having her around. We were never particularly close as children as, due to the gaps in our ages, we all played with different circles of friends. I suppose, as children, we found it annoying to have the 'little sister' or 'big brother' hanging around. I was a bit wild and my brother would delight in dampening my enthusiasm by reminding me that he would tell Mum and Dad on me if I didn't behave.

I remember being a very happy child. Thurles was a very safe place to live and everybody knew everybody else. I would spend all my days out playing with all the other children. Once I got up in the morning, I would be out of the house and gone for the whole day. I would go to friends' houses and we would go out and play simple games that could last for hours. I would only go home for lunch or dinner and even that, to me, was a nuisance because I didn't want to miss anything.

Like everybody in Ireland in the 1960s, our life was very simple and we didn't have a lot of material things, but my parents always made a huge effort. Christmas in particular was always very special to me. My mother would buy everything on the quiet and when Christmas Eve came, we would want to go to bed at some ridiculous time like six o'clock in the evening because we wanted Christmas Day to arrive as soon as possible. The other reason was because Mum did nothing to the house until we were in bed on Christmas Eve. Then she would put up the Christmas tree and all the decorations and the paper chains across the ceiling, as we did in those days, and put the presents under the tree. The turkey would be stuffed and the vegetables would be prepared. When we awoke on Christmas morning, we would tear down the stairs into the sitting room and there it would be: Christmas would have arrived magically overnight. It was a sight to behold. I loved the way she did that. It literally was as if someone had sprinkled fairy dust on the house while we were asleep. I never thought about the work that must have gone into that and how late Mum must have had to stay up to get it all done. Like many men at the time, my father was never very hands-on when it came to the children or the house and so Mum would have had to do all of the work herself.

Every year from about the age of five I would ask for a bike from Santa. It was a huge thing in the Sixties to get a bike for Christmas. I never did get the bike, but it didn't seem to matter. Whatever I got was always the most fantastic thing ever. I found out about Santa's real identity when I was ten years old and Christmas has never been the same since. After that, there were no toys and it was always something that you needed, like a coat or a pair of boots. What a reality check that was. When my own children were young, I did the same thing as Mum one Christmas and the kids really enjoyed it, but they *were* very young: as they got older, the pressure to put up a tree earlier and earlier soon put a stop to the tradition.

As I said, I was a bit wild when I was young, but in a very innocent way. Like any other child, I would push the boundaries with my mum and come home later than I was allowed. I would be terrified about how I would be punished but, as far as I was concerned, it was worth it because the *craic* was too good and I worried that I would have missed something otherwise. I started smoking at the tender age of fourteen because it was a cool thing to do. I felt so grown-up as I exhaled the smoke, trying to make rings and various shapes with my mouth. At that time, there was a local shop near the school that used to sell single cigarettes – imagine that nowadays? I think it was two pence for a 'fag', as we used to call it. However, if you managed to get a whole box of ten, you were really cool.

I always went around in a group. There were maybe three or four of us. Sometimes we would rob apple orchards and then set up a fire and cook the apples and eat them. Afterwards I would go home, stinking of bonfire smoke and Mum would go mad. I can't blame her when I think about it because there was no such thing as a washing machine and everything was done by hand. We had no running hot water in the early days and once a week, Mum would boil pots and pots of water to fill the bath and then we would take turns washing ourselves before we ran in front of the fire to warm ourselves up. There was no central heating then and all the heat in the house came from the fireplace. I loved the open fire and still do to this day. There is something magical about staring into the flames of an open fire. Some people think that they are dirty and too much bother, but not me. I still have, and always will have, an open fire in my house.

Mum did get a 'twin tub', as they were called, a few years later, which consisted of a washer and separate spinner in one machine. You had to fill the machine manually and one side washed the clothes and the other side spun them afterwards. That was considered really posh in those days!

In the summertime we would walk a couple of miles to Lady's Well on the River Suir, where we all used to hang out and swim or just relax in the sun. It was fantastic because there was a deep area where you could dive, a medium-depth area where you could swim, and a shallow area for children to paddle. All the parents used to sit on the riverbank and they would have sandwiches and tea so that we could spend the day there. A free-flowing river can be pretty cold, but I can never remember that being a problem, even though my mother would insist on me coming out of the water because I was cold and I would insist that I was fine, even though my lips and skin were purple and I couldn't stop shivering. We had fantastic carefree days, when the summers seemed longer, brighter and hotter. Perhaps these summers exist only in my memory, but I loved my life as a child and I feel sorry for my own children that the simplicity of those days was well gone by the time they arrived in the world.

*

One of the fond memories I have of my childhood was that my mother was always at home. There were very few days when I would come home from school that she wasn't there. So much so, that if she wasn't, I would be really upset with her. It was so comforting to arrive home after school and Mum would be there waiting for us. We always came home at lunchtime, when we would have our main meal of the day and in the evening, when we would have our tea, which might just consist of tea, bread and butter with jam and maybe an apple tart. I loved my mum's apple tarts! It was very reassuring and home really felt like home. I sometimes think that my children and many others missed out on that, but I suppose they don't know what it was like, so they don't miss it.

I started school in September 1965 at the tender age of five. I went to the Presentation Convent in Thurles, which was run almost totally by nuns at the time and I remained there until I left school in 1977. I enjoyed school and I particularly liked the social aspect of it. I liked to be funny and to try and make people laugh. I wouldn't say I was very clever, as I found it very difficult to study and concentrate, but I was a bright child and had a lot of common sense. I never had very high grades at school, but they were enough to get by on.

My love of music began at school, where I particularly loved it as a subject and I studied musicianship as part of my Intermediate Certificate, which I took in 1975. I remember learning about Impressionist music, the music of composers like Debussy and Ravel, and I loved it when the teacher would play some classical piece and ask us to close our eyes and imagine what we saw. We learned how to write music and all about manuscripts, notes and timing. I did very well in my exams and wanted to continue to take music for my Leaving Certificate in 1977.

I was so keen that I even tried to learn a few instruments, but that never worked out. First, I took piano lessons. Initially, I enjoyed it and every day after school I would go to the music rooms to practise my scales (I don't think I ever got past the scales stage!). Once a week, we would have to play the scales over and over on a one-to-one basis with the teacher to see how well we had been practising. If we played a note wrong, she would hit us on our knuckles with the side of a ruler and reprimand us. After a few months, I'd had enough of that nonsense and gave up the piano as a bad job. I just didn't think that all that hard work was worth the pain of being regularly hit with the side of a ruler and I was fed up to the back teeth with playing scales.

When I think of it now, it really was a crazy thing to do, to rap us on the knuckles, not least because it certainly did nothing to encourage me to play. Also, knuckles are a very important part of a pianist's hands and who knows what damage could have been inflicted on them. Apart from all that, patience was definitely not my forte because I thought I would be playing Rachmaninov after my fifth lesson!

The second instrument I attempted was the violin. I desperately wanted to be a part of music in whatever form it would take, but again, it was a bit of a disaster: I only got as far as playing 'Twinkle, Twinkle Little Star', before I had a fight with one of the other students and hit her with the bow, which snapped the head off. As the instrument was school property and I had behaved in such an unladylike manner, I was thrown out of the orchestra.

Finally, I went to the local brass band to see if there were any vacancies. I was in luck as they needed someone to play the trombone. Hmm . . . not really the romantic instrument I had visualized myself playing and entertaining an audience with. Once again, my giddiness got the better of me when, on my fifth week, I was messing with one of the lads and I split my lip on the trombone and couldn't play for the next six weeks, by which time the idea of marching up and down the town in the freezing cold just didn't appeal to me any more.

That was the end of my attempts to learn an instrument, but I still wanted music to be part of my life. The convent had very good facilities for music and sports, even in the 1960s, but sadly, in those days, we did not have career guidance counsellors and our subject choices were left pretty much up to ourselves. I was told by a friend that I couldn't do music for my Leaving Certificate if I didn't have an instrument, which, as you now know, I didn't. I was so disappointed that I had to give it up, but I thought I had no choice. I later discovered that I could have used my voice as an instrument, but it was too late for me. I suppose what surprises me now is that nobody questioned why I gave up a subject I was good at and obviously enjoyed. If the teachers had questioned me, I would have realized that I could continue with music and who knows how that might have changed my future.

Certainly, at that time, music was everything to me. I remember at the start of secondary school, we were all gathered in the Assembly Hall one day, so that the nuns could decide who was good enough to sing in the choir. We all sat in the hall, chatting away, while one nun sat at a piano at the top and each girl had to go up and sing a piece of music. Everyone who went up was very quiet and you could barely hear them singing. When it was my turn, I went to the top of the hall and belted out a classic song called, 'It's Too Late Baby', by Carole King, whom I loved at the time. I think when I started singing I even surprised myself at how strong my voice was. Everyone stopped and stared and I was mortified! I did get into the choir and that was my first real experience of singing and I loved the way it made me feel.

I suppose if I had any regrets in my life, it would be that I did nothing about my love of music at that time. The problem was that I just didn't know how to go about it. I mean, how do you suddenly decide to be a singer? Where do you go? Nowadays, they have programmes on TV like *The X Factor* or *Britain's Got Talent*, but there was nothing like that when I was growing up. Another problem was my confidence. Even though I loved singing, I just didn't believe I was good enough. That belief in yourself is so important and that is why I tell my children: everything is possible if you want it badly enough. I wanted it, but I didn't believe it was possible. Perhaps my life might have turned out differently if I had pursued singing, but that's something I will never know. I needed to accept and to believe in myself before anything like that could happen.

I got another chance to take to the stage and to sing when the school staged 'Joseph and the Amazing Technicolor Dreamcoat', a very popular musical at the time. As I was attending an all-girls' Catholic school, there were no boys for any of the roles and we could audition for any part. I was delighted when I was chosen to play the part of Joseph. It was the best experience I had ever had at that stage in my life. Singing songs made me feel so happy. I have to admit that standing in front of an audience was a bit scary. I didn't really enjoy that part so much and to this day, I still get very nervous on stage, but I just loved the singing part. When I eventually recorded my own album, I loved being in the studio where no one was watching me and I was lost in a world of my own with the headphones on. If I forgot the words it didn't matter because I could start again.

Shortly after that, in 1975, the Thurles Musical Society, of which I was a member, decided to stage the musical 'Jesus Christ Superstar'. We were one of the first amateur musical groups in Ireland to do this production and we had to get special permission from Tim Rice and Andrew Lloyd Webber, who wrote the musical, at the time. Anyone from the town who was interested was asked to attend auditions and there was a lot of excitement about it. Someone had heard me in 'Joseph' and said that I should go along. I tried out for the part of Mary Magdalene and was delighted when I was successful.

There were months of rehearsals in the run-up to the big night, and the production ran for five nights in the Premier Hall in Thurles. Once again, I was in heaven! I can honestly say that it was one of the best periods in my life: I was carefree, happy and fulfilled. I looked forward to the rehearsals every week and the socializing that went with it, as well as to the performances. The show was such a huge success that we decided to do it the following year for another five nights. After that, we staged the musical 'Hair', which was a very forward-thinking production for a small town in Ireland in 1976! Once again, I had one of the lead roles and was totally immersed in everything about it for that summer.

Even though music filled my life at that time, I never once thought about singing as a career. It just never occurred to me. I had no connections in the business and I knew nobody who had followed that life. To me, it was just something that you did for fun or as a hobby. I just didn't see that it was something at which you could make a living. Also, I don't think my father would have been too happy if I had come home and said I was going to sing for a career. He wanted us to have stable wages coming in every week, holiday and sick pay and maybe even a pension.

Music also led me to my first romance and was very much the 'soundtrack' to my teenage years. There was a band in Thurles at that time called Pyramid and they were doing the musical score for the production of 'Jesus Christ Superstar'. I was fifteen at the time and they were all in their early twenties, which seemed so grown-up and mature to me. I was smitten with the bass player and it wasn't long before we were an item. This meant that I was able to go to their rehearsals and be with them any time they played a gig. I loved being part of the music scene, even as a spectator. My boyfriend, whose name I shall leave out for fear I might embarrass him, was a very kind and gentle man and we got on very well and became really good friends. We were together for three years and I am very glad that my first encounter with love and the opposite sex was such a positive one.

At the time I thought I would end up marrying him because that's what you did. You went to school, got your education, met a partner, got married and had your family. Simple as that. He was my first love because it was the first time that I experienced genuine caring and interest in me, outside of my family, and, of course, we had the love of music in common. I remember that my mother wasn't happy that I was seeing a guy five years older than me. I suppose she thought he would corrupt me in some way, but it couldn't have been further from the truth. All the guys in the band were very caring, decent blokes who would look out for you and always insist that you were seen home if you were out late at night.

Another close friend of mine at the time started seeing the lead guitar player, so now I had someone to hang out with and talk to at school and socially who understood what it was like – the band were so talented, writing their own numbers as well as doing covers, and any time I went to hear them playing, I was elated. That might sound a bit strong, but it's the truth. I genuinely felt so happy and care-free and lost in the music. I was also the band's biggest fan: I had huge respect for them and their talents. I couldn't understand why they hadn't made it in Ireland and I believed that everyone should know about them and how good they were.

A few years back, I returned to Thurles as I'd heard they

were having a reunion gig and once they started playing, I was back there, back to the 1970s, those innocent times when I had my whole life ahead of me. The band sounded as good to me as they always had. Of course, they all looked different, as did I, and they had wives and families that I knew little of, but it was a great night and wonderful to forget everything that had happened in the nearly thirty years since I had last seen them together. Just for a little while, I felt sixteen all over again!

Like many fathers at the time, Dad was very strict and he would not have approved of my boyfriend because he was older and he had long hair and played in a band. Oh no, my father would have wanted a lawyer, doctor or businessman for me, even though I was only fifteen. As far as Dad was concerned, until I reached the age of eighteen, I was to do everything I was told. The day after my eighteenth birthday, I could do as I pleased.

Because I was a bit of a live wire as a teenager, this sometimes got me into hot water. One night in particular, there was a gig in town and Pyramid were playing. I desperately wanted to go. Mum was easy to persuade about these things, but Dad was another matter. I knew he wouldn't let me go, as the gig finished at one a.m. and I was barely allowed to go to the disco that finished at eleven p.m., never mind going to see a band until one in the morning. I decided that I would wait until Mum and Dad were in bed and then I would make my escape through the bedroom window. It's amazing how determined you can be when you want something badly.

I waited and waited until I felt they were asleep, which, by this time, was about a quarter past midnight. I knew it would take me a good twenty minutes to get to the venue if I ran fast enough, but I didn't care. I just had to get there, in case I might miss something. Luckily, we lived in a bungalow, so I opened my bedroom window, slowly stepped out and ran like hell until I reached the venue. It was a quarter to one at this stage, so I only had fifteen minutes before the gig was over, but I didn't care. I was there and that's all that mattered. I saw who was shifting who (shifting was the term we used in the 70s, where snogging or kissing is now used) who fell out with who and everything I felt I needed to know to be a finger-on-the-pulse kind of girl on the social scene. Then it was time to go home.

It had started to rain very heavily, but I meandered slowly home digesting all that I had seen. I arrived back at my house at about two a.m. and all was quiet. Great. Another successful night on the town (this was about the third time I had tried this) and home without anyone being any the wiser. How wrong I was. I opened the bedroom window and climbed up on the window sill. I stepped over the window sill and put my feet on the bedroom floor. Then it happened . . . On my window sill I had all my bottles of 'things' a young girl had at the time, like 4711 eau de Cologne, Anne French cleansing lotion, bottles of nail varnish, that kind of thing. As I'd climbed in the window, my coat had brushed against all the bottles and pulled them down, clattering and clanging off the radiator and onto the floor. The noise was unbelievable. Oh, bugger! I thought. What to do now? I knew my parents would have heard the noise because it was so loud, so I decided to jump into bed fully clothed and pretend that I was asleep. This was ridiculous as my hair was soaking wet and the window was still open. Next thing, the bedroom light went on and there my dad stood, in his pyjama pants, wanting to know what the hell was going on. Worse still, he demanded to know who had been in my bedroom. It's funny how parents' imaginations can overtake reality. I was horrified, to say the least. At this stage, I was a virgin and really very innocent when it came to sex. I was a fantastic kisser, or so I thought anyway, because kissing was everything at that time. You could experience so many wonderful feelings just by kissing. You could be playful, serious, sad, bold and any number of things through your kissing. It was wonderful. As for the other, it had never crossed my mind. I was too scared of becoming pregnant to let any guy near me. I knew so little about it really, like many Irish girls at the time. As far as I was concerned, if I stood naked with a naked man beside me and he touched me, I could be pregnant! Those little pests would somehow manage to escape the man's private parts and travel, Gods knows how, up inside me without me even knowing. And then my father would really kill me. No, kissing was enough for me, thank you.

I desperately tried to explain to Dad that that was not the case: no man had been in my bed. I had been out, but no one had been in. He was so angry, he threatened to hit me with his belt (something he had never done before), but my mum came in and defused the situation, persuading him to calm down. I think he believed me because I was lying in the bed with soaking wet hair! I had been given a watch for Christmas and he took it off me as a punishment, telling me that I didn't deserve it and that when I had proved that I could be trusted again, I could have the watch back. The fact that I had disappointed him hurt very much and I was sorry that he hadn't slapped me instead. It would have been over and done with, but I had a constant reminder now in the fact that my watch had been taken from me. I got it back about five months later. Obviously, I never tried that trick again.

I freely admit that I was a bundle of energy as a teenager. I was always on the go and I could never sit still. I never read a book or spent any time sitting on my own. I didn't like that. I wanted to be out with people all the time. I was very thin and seemed to have an excessive amount of nervous energy. As I said earlier, I was a bit of a tomboy so I liked to do all the things that the boys did. I had no idea how to flirt with a guy; in fact, I suppose flirting never really crossed my mind. I had no idea about fashion or no real interest in it. I find it amazing that my daughter has a wonderful sense of style and fashion and can throw anything together and look stunning. She certainly didn't get that from me! I didn't wear make-up or even have a handbag until I was nineteen and living in London. I only wore make-up then because I thought I had to. Everybody else wore it and I would have looked odd without at least a bit of mascara and lipstick.

As I said earlier, I became a smoker when I was fourteen.

Like a lot of teenagers, I wanted to try smoking because all the older ones were doing it. I wanted to be popular with everyone and I remember for a period my mother used to look after my grandmother's shop that sold confectionery and cigarettes. Every now and then I would take a packet of cigarettes from the shop without my parents knowing and I would go to meet up with my friends feeling ever so grown-up because I had a whole pack of cigarettes. Kudos! The cigarettes would get shared amongst everyone and we would all feel like grown-ups for the evening. How naïve we were. I suppose, like everyone starting out, I had to be 'taught' how to smoke and how to hold the cigarette properly. I didn't want to look like a novice so one of my more experienced friends would take a pull and inhale it and I would watch her and try to copy her. The first few times I coughed liked crazy and it felt awful, but I had to keep going until I looked like a real pro. We would all hang out in a small café in the town where they had a jukebox and we would all congregate in the evenings. Most of us didn't have any money, so we would try and scrape together the price of a bag of chips and a Coke and we would all sit in the café and listen to music while we shared our meal.

*

My mum and dad moved to Dublin in 1976 when I was going into my Leaving Certificate year, so they decided that I should go into boarding school at the Presentation Convent for my final year. Being in boarding school was quite restricting, but I really enjoyed the experience, though I still managed to get up to mischief at times. We were only allowed to go home for the holidays, but we could go out on Sunday afternoons if a member of our family came to collect us. Most of the other boarders in the school were not from the town, which made it a little easier for them to settle. Because I had been a day pupil all of my life and I knew everybody in the town, I wanted to get out and see my friends as much as I could. So, when Sunday afternoons came, I would tell the nun in charge that my parents or aunt or whoever had come for me and were in a terrible rush and that I could not find them to get permission to go. That usually worked and I would skip off out to one of my friend's houses for the day. Once I had finished my Leaving Certificate examination, I moved to Dublin because that's where the family was at that stage.

Looking back, I had a very happy childhood and the memories I have of growing up in Thurles will always be good ones that will stay with me forever. In Thurles, I discovered that I loved music, I had a group of great friends and I came from a loving family, all of which would sustain me over the coming years. I was also lucky, I think, to have a great deal of freedom. Even though Ireland at the time was a very different place, looking back, they were such innocent times.

Chapter 3

MUM AND DAD

If my childhood growing up in rural Ireland made me the person I am today, my parents have played an even bigger role in my life. I am very like my father and am told this on a regular basis. When I was younger, it bothered me because I didn't like him very much and I just couldn't relate to him. I did not see myself as being similar to him and I certainly didn't want to be! But now, I'm grateful for the similarity.

My dad passed away very suddenly after a fall on 15 October 2013. I miss him dearly and I am very grateful that he lived long enough for me to get to know him as an adult. If that had not happened, I would have greatly misjudged the man my father was.

My mother is my hero: she has been my rock throughout my life, a source of support and strength when I've needed her. She was always there when I was growing up and, like so many Irish mothers, she did everything for her family. Without Mum and Dad, I wouldn't be the person I am today.

Having said that, family life isn't always easy, as so many of you will know. Dad was an old-fashioned father in so many ways and so different at home. Out in the world, he was well liked by everyone. He was outgoing and entertaining and loved to be the centre of attention when he was socializing. He was involved in lots of things and everything he did, he did to the absolute best of his ability. When he was young, he cycled for Tipperary and won many medals. He played golf off a handicap of four. He was a member of the Thurles Operatic Society and often played the part of the comedian, which suited him to a tee! I credit Dad with my love of music and performing.

Dad was also a great sailor and every summer he would sail around Ireland with like-minded friends, having the time of his life along the way. Dad was more of a home-grown sailor, though, even though he'd studied for, and got, his captain's licence. What I mean by that is that he was rough and ready. The first boat I remember him sailing was a Galway hooker. A beautiful boat, but by no means fancy: in spite of their lovely red sails, Galway hookers are working boats. You can be sure that if you ever went on that boat with Dad, you would emerge with bits of tar stuck to your clothes here and there, and there was no toilet, so it was a case of doing your business in a bucket and throwing it overboard. Not the kind of antics you would expect to see in the yacht clubs in Dún Laoghaire.

Sailing always involved drinking and my father could do that very well. Don't get me wrong, he was a very attentive sailor and would never take a drink until the sailing day was over. He would leave one port in the morning, sail all day until he arrived at the next and then it would be into the pub to 'give it a lash' as he would say. We had a caravan in Spiddal, Co. Galway, and he moored his boat at the pier there, so most of his sailing was around Connemara and Mayo, up the coast to Donegal. There always seemed to be live traditional Irish music in the pubs on the coast in those days. It was brilliant. When we went with him, we'd arrive in a port, we would have a meal and then we'd go to the pub and listen to the music and entertain ourselves in whatever way we could, while dad was entertaining everyone else with his antics. At the end of the night, we'd head back to the caravan and Mum would put on the frying pan and dish up a big fry to whomever Dad decided to bring with him that night. I would be put to bed, but I loved to lie there and listen to the stories, the arguments and the songs people would sing.

Dad spent every last penny and effort getting his beloved Galway hooker into the best shape possible. He loved that boat. However, one year, not long after he had finished restoring the boat, there was a huge storm and Dad arrived down to the pier in Spiddal the morning after to see half of the hooker on the beach and the other half in bits floating in the water. I felt so sorry for Dad that day. He was distraught. After that, he had a concrete boat (I know it sounds crazy, but it's true. A big lump of concrete floating in the water!) He called that *The Concrete Jungle* and we had many happy times in that boat, too. Eventually, he sailed his small yacht from Dublin to Tenerife with a couple of his friends and had some very interesting stories to tell when he returned.

At home, though, my dad was a very different man. When I was young and I went to my friends' houses, their parents would ask who I was 'belonging to', in the usual Irish way. 'Ah, you're Tom Roche's daughter. He's a great man,' would usually be the response when I told them. I could never understand it as I thought they must be mistaking him for someone else. At home he was a very different man. He was very intolerant of children and he never really talked to me or my siblings about anything. He never seemed interested in us. I was also afraid of him as he was very aggressive in his manner with us. He was very quick to judge when you did something he didn't approve of. As he was away a lot of the time, my mother would use him as a threat to get us to behave. As I said before, sometimes your imagination is worse than reality as I would always assume that he would punish us physically, which was never the case. However, the threat was always there in my mind.

My mother was eighteen when she married and my father was twenty. They were just children really. That explains so much that I didn't understand when I was young. There were three of us by the time Mum was twenty-three and Dad was twenty-five. I cannot begin to imagine what that must have been like at the time, but they just got on with it. Or, if I'm honest, I should say Mum got on with it and Dad just got on. What I mean by that is, Mum was left with the rearing, while Dad continued to be a 'lad'. I don't think he understood what it meant to be a parent, but I think that was fairly par for the course in those days.

Mum did everything – and I mean everything. She cooked, cleaned, shopped and did the gardening. She brought us to school and collected us. She did any repairs that needed doing in the house and she was a mean wall-paperer. Dad had no interest in any of it. As long as the house provided a roof over his head then he was happy. Mum, on the other hand, was a very proud person and she liked everything to be proper. The house was always spotless and welcoming and homely. They didn't have much as a young couple, but I never knew that and it never showed. As we got older, Mum worked in a bakery, but regardless of what was going on in her life and how busy she was, the dinner was always on the table when my dad came home. That was expected of her and he would not have been happy if it was any other way. Dad, on the other hand, had a good time. As well as his golf and sailing, he played in a band, he was in the operatic society and he went out regularly for a few drinks with his friends.

Dad found it very hard to express any kind of affection at all. He never put his arms around us as children or told us he loved us. He would criticize everything from our posture to our diction, but you never got a 'well done' from him. He just couldn't say it. I know there were times when he wanted to say something encouraging, but it was as if the words got stuck in his throat. I suppose we all bring our children up influenced by the way in which we were brought up ourselves and Dad's father had been a strong disciplinarian. Dad probably thought that that was how a father should be with his children. He demanded respect, whereas nowadays, I want to earn the respect of my children. His parents had also been very strict and he never heard those words of encouragement while he was growing up, so perhaps that explains it. I believe it is our duty as parents to show our children how to love and to express love and to feel confident as people and if it hasn't been practised while they are growing up, then how are they supposed to learn? Luckily, my mother was very affectionate so I got a lot of loving from her.

I can remember my father's behaviour very clearly on a few occasions. These stand out because they affected me so much at the time. When I was about four or five, he asked me to clean his shoes for him. I was really happy that he'd asked me because that meant that I might be able to impress him and he might say something really nice to me to make me feel loved. I cleaned those shoes to within an inch of my life and I thought I had done a great job. When

I gave him the shoes back, with a big grin on my face, he told me they weren't good enough and to do them again. I was devastated because I knew that I had done the very best I could and I didn't know what else to do. Isn't it amazing how something as trivial as that could make such an impression on a child that it has stuck with me for all these years? We don't realize what effect a thoughtless remark can have on a child.

Another time I remember very vividly was when I got the lead female role in 'Jesus Christ Superstar'. I was delighted with myself and I was sure Mum and Dad would be really proud. I couldn't believe my luck when Dad agreed to come and see the production because everybody in the town was talking about how good it was, so I guess he thought he should go. He watched the show and as it was the last show of the run, I was presented with a huge bouquet of flowers afterwards. I walked down to Mum and Dad holding my flowers, feeling as if I was on cloud nine and expecting: 'Well done, that was great.' Instead, what I actually got was: 'Hmm … your diction could have been better'! Talk about bursting your bubble. It seemed that nothing I did could please him.

This, of course, was only my perception of him through young, naïve eyes. I know now that my father was indeed very proud of me, but he couldn't say those words. He thought that constructive criticism was what I needed and he just wanted to help me to do better the next time. I know where he was coming from, but it is so important to tell your children that you are proud of them and that they have done well, even if they're not perfect. I guess most dads were like that in those days. I have lots of friends whose fathers were similar. It was just how things were and you had to put up with it. I know I have gone overboard telling my children that they are great, and yet I can hear my father talking as I tell them how they could improve! It's very hard to break away from what you have been brought up with. Once I had my own children, I understood more clearly what my father was trying to do. I'm not saying he was right or wrong, just that I now understand why he behaved as he did.

While my upbringing definitely affected my own life and the way I brought my children up, in some ways, I have gone the opposite way to my dad. I never wanted them to feel the way I did about my father as a child. I wanted to bring up my children so that they are not afraid to say, 'I love you, Mum' and vice-versa, or to put their arms around me and have a good cuddle. I constantly tell them I love them and that I'm proud of them. All I ever want for my children is to be happy and confident and to be able to provide for themselves and for their families. After that, I don't care if they are road sweepers or doctors. I don't want my children to be doing something that stresses them out for years on end just so that I can boast about how well they've done. I see many parents like that. Status is everything to them. I believe that you should rear your children to be happy, confident people and then let them go, to experience their own lives and to make their own mistakes. I'm always there for my children and they know that, but I don't interfere in their lives. Life is very short and it is so important that they are true to themselves, work hard at whatever it is they choose and let everything else just happen.

My father taught me to be independent and feisty and to work hard at everything I did. For that I am very grateful and I certainly know that I would not have got on as well in life without his influence. He didn't do that deliberately though, that was just how I turned out because of the way he behaved towards me. They are the good points. However, I also grew up feeling unloved and unworthy and with a distorted need for a man to show me love. I desperately wanted my father to show me love: he did, of course, love me, but I never felt it.

When I left home in the 1970s to go to London, I didn't come home very often, maybe once a year. Dad would pick me up from the boat at Dun Laoghaire and all he would say would be, 'How are ya?' That's it. No hug, no kiss and certainly no conversation. He wouldn't ask me what I was doing or anything about my life. I would spend the journey home in the car feeling very uncomfortable and asking trivial questions just to pass the time. 'How's Mum?' 'Fine.' 'How's work?' 'Grand.' Always one-word answers. I would be dying to get to the front door of the house to see Mum, when I would fully relax and feel I was at home.

One day, though, Dad surprised me. It was the day I got married to my first husband, Raymond. I was twenty-six years old and on the way to the church in the bridal car, with Dad on my right-hand side. He caught my hand, but kept looking straight ahead and he said, 'You do know that I love you.' I was flabbergasted, to say the least. I felt such a mix of emotions. On the one hand, I was absolutely delighted. I felt so happy that he had finally said those words to me and at the same time I wanted to scream: 'NO. OF COURSE I DIDN'T KNOW. YOU NEVER TOLD ME.' What I actually said, without looking at him either, was, 'Yes.' That was it. I couldn't say another word. Looking back now, I know how hard it must have been for him to say those words and they mean so much more because of that.

As we got older, I would tell Dad that I loved him in a jokey kind of way, partly because I knew it made him uncomfortable and mostly because I knew he did, in fact, love to hear it, even if he couldn't say it himself. He might say, 'Ah, that's a load of old nonsense! You don't need to tell people you love them. They should know!' But actually, people do need to hear it as well, especially when they are children. I knew my Dad loved me, but I am sad that I didn't know it as a child.

As I look back on his life, I feel sorry for my father that he missed out on so much. Obviously I am not talking about his social life, which couldn't have been better, but from an emotional and family point of view. He had a wonderful wife, who treated him like a king and four children who have turned out to be pretty decent people, if I say so myself, but he just couldn't connect with us as children. I could never talk to Dad about anything and I am glad that my children are open and honest with me. I feel very privileged that they are in my life.

Myself and my brother and sisters appreciated Dad as we got older and I got to really enjoy the person he was and to see his strengths, which I had a lot of admiration for. I suppose it can take a long time to fully understand anyone. Your perception of someone also depends on what stage you are at in your life. I said at the beginning of this chapter that I am glad that Dad lived long enough for us both to get to know each other properly because if Dad had died when I was younger, I really wouldn't have had much regard for him. How wrong that would have been. You really do need to walk in someone else's shoes to understand them.

Over the last twelve years, I have spent a lot of time with my mum and dad. That is, in part, down to Daniel. He was absolutely wonderful with them from the beginning. He always included them in everything we did. If we were going out for dinner, he would say, 'Ask your mum and dad if they want to come'. At first, I thought it was very strange because it wouldn't have been something I would generally do, but Daniel made it feel very natural. Then it became the norm. They were almost like our friends and the age difference didn't matter. My parents are great fun and very open-minded, so we all got on very well. Before Dad's death, we went on holidays together several times. Mum and Dad bought a home in Tenerife in 1991 and because Daniel and I have a holiday home there, we saw them a lot. They used to spend most of the year on the island, but

Mum will spend most of her time in Ireland now that Dad is gone, apart from a few weeks in the winter. We want to keep her here and look after her. I don't like the idea of her being all on her own so far away.

Daniel loves playing cards and Mum and Dad did too, so we used to go to their place regularly for a few games. I ended up not enjoying it because Daniel and I would always end up fighting, so I stopped going. Daniel is very competitive when it comes to cards or golf! He would surprise most people with how seriously he takes challenges. Daniel, however, continued to play cards with my parents whenever he could and now that Dad is gone, he still plays the odd game with Mum.

Dad looked after our house in Tenerife and it was reassuring to know that he would do any repairs that were necessary and just generally keep an eye on it. Any time friends were arriving in Tenerife, he would volunteer to pick them up and drop them off at the airport. I have been out there a couple of times since he died and it feels very strange not having him there to greet me. In the complex where my parents have a holiday home, people always came to Dad if something needed to be fixed. It didn't matter if it was the television or the toilet, he could sort it. However, Mum always had to get on to him to do things in his own house. How many men do you know like that?! He would do anything to help someone else out.

I remember so well the moment my sister rang me to tell me that Dad had had a fall in Tenerife. It was Saturday morning 12 October 2013 and I was sitting in my apartment in Dublin. I had had my second round of chemo on 3 October, so I was just beginning to feel like a human again. My mother, who was staying with me while I went through the chemo, was still in bed. I was on a Skype call to my brother, Michael, in England, when my mobile phone rang. My daughter Siobhán was at the apartment with her boyfriend, Gavin, and she answered the phone. She told me it was my sister, Jo. 'Tell her I'll call her back,' I said, as I was still talking to Michael. To my surprise, Siobhán insisted that it was urgent and that Jo needed to talk to me straight away. That is very unusual in our household. When I took the phone, Jo told me that Dad was in hospital in a critical condition after having a fall. I was in complete shock and I let a roar out of me. I knew by the tone of Jo's voice that it was very serious.

I have never seen my father in hospital, or even sick. He was a very healthy man. The first thing I wanted to do was to get out to Tenerife to see what the story was. How serious was it? Would he recover? Could they operate? What state was he in? Was he dying? All these questions were running through my mind. I was in turmoil. Then there was Mum. I had no idea what I would say to her. She has been with my father since she was eighteen years old and she is now seventy-six. That's fifty-eight years. I dreaded having to tell her and I had no idea how to do it.

I went into the bedroom, where she was still fast asleep and I hesitated for a moment, unsure whether to tell her straight away or wait for her to get up. There was simply no easy way to tell her. However, I am not very good at hiding things and you have to remember that I was in shock, too. I decided that I would tell her while she was lying down just in case she might collapse. I regret that now because all Mum saw when she awoke was my face peering down at her, telling her the worst possible news. She had only just woken up, God love her.

Mum was very calm, but obviously shocked. When I told my mother I had cancer, she reacted in the same way. I suppose that's her way of coping. It's almost as if she closes down and lets none of her emotions out, just in case they overwhelm her.

We got ourselves together in a bit of a panic and Gavin got on the computer and managed to book a couple of seats on a flight to Tenerife, leaving at two that afternoon. That was a horrible journey because we didn't know what to expect when we got there. I wondered if he would be dead already, or brain damaged and I worried about how Mum would react when she saw him. Would we have a chance to say goodbye, I worried, or was this it? I had wondered from time to time, as I suppose we all do, how and when I would lose my parents from my life. Who would go first? Who would do better without the other and now all these questions were going round and round in my head. I felt like we were in limbo up there in the air and I wondered if things had progressed on the ground and if there had been any developments. It was agony not knowing anything and not being able to contact anyone for those four hours.

When we arrived in Tenerife at eight o'clock that night, we went straight to Hospiten Sur, or the Green Clinic as it's also known. We went to the intensive care unit, which had about ten beds in it all in a row. Dad was in the second bed from the door and Mum and I both broke down when we saw him. Here was the big, strong man that I knew lying there, totally motionless, with all these tubes coming out of his mouth to breathe for him. I kissed his forehead and rubbed his face and did all the things that I could never have done when he was conscious. I held his hand and fixed his hair and whispered that I loved him very much in his ear. He was so still. It was as if he was already dead, but the machine was keeping him alive. He didn't look dead, thank God – in fact, he looked just as he always had. Mum was sobbing quietly and was as dignified as always, but trying desperately to contain her emotions. She is a very proud person and would take whatever is thrown her way in a dignified manner. The people in the beds around my father were all conscious and it was difficult for us as we didn't have any privacy.

We asked to speak to a doctor to find out what the story was as we knew nothing other than the fact that he was unconscious. We didn't know if it was an induced coma or a natural coma. We didn't know if he could be operated on or needed airlifting somewhere else. We had so many questions to which we needed answers. Unfortunately, in spite of our pleas, there was no-one available until the following morning. Reluctantly we had to leave, still knowing nothing about his condition. I just wanted to get him out of there back to Ireland because at least then we might get a clearer understanding of what was happening.

The next morning, the doctor came to the unit at eleven

and started at the top of the ward working with an interpreter and speaking to each patient and family about their relative's condition. The doctor eventually reached our bed and told us that Dad was in a very critical condition and that he had a fractured skull and a bleed and that his brain was very swollen. In short, there was no hope for him. I was devastated. This was it. My father was going to die. Right out of the blue, with no warning whatsoever. Mum was just numb. In my distressed state, it just seemed to me that the doctors were very cold and, of course, the language barrier didn't help to soften the blow of the news.

Every time we visited Dad over the following days, he was in exactly the same condition. There was no movement whatsoever and this took its toll on Mum. She would be OK when she arrived at the hospital, but every time she saw Dad, she would break down. The rest of the family were already on their way, but my younger sister Moira, who lives in New Zealand, had a long journey ahead of her. We knew that there was no hope and we just wanted it to end. It was torture. As each member of the family arrived, the torture continued. After Moira had made it in from New Zealand, we asked if the machine could be switched off because it was obvious he was never going to recover and we didn't want him to suffer any longer. We were told that as he was in an induced coma, he would have to be in a natural coma for at least twenty-four hours before they could do a brain-stem test to see if there was any activity. That test was done on Tuesday morning and it showed that Dad had no brain activity whatsoever. We decided to switch the machine off at six o'clock that evening.

When we had first realized that Dad was not going to recover, we asked if he could be moved into a private room so that we could say our goodbyes, but that was not possible. We stood by his bed, which was an arm's length from the next bed with the bustle of the intensive care unit going on around us, and we all cried. It was a horrible way to say goodbye. The woman in the bed next to Dad was from another country and she was eating her dinner and telling us not to cry. The man on the other side was naked, lying on his side with his bottom on display. I asked the nurse to please cover him up, as it just felt so wrong for my father's last hours on this earth and for his family trying to say goodbye. We were all distraught.

The time came and the doctor came to switch the machine off. What they actually do is remove the tubes and wait for things to take their course. The doctor said it could be ten minutes or two hours. It was awful waiting and watching the machine as his blood pressure went lower and lower. I held his hand the whole time and told him that we would look after Mum and that he could go peacefully. His grandchildren were at the hospital and some close friends of Dad's, but only his children were allowed to be at his bedside while he slipped away. The others were in the corridor sobbing their hearts out.

Luckily Daniel stayed with us and he was a wonderful comfort to us. We didn't know what to do, but Daniel started praying and we joined in as the life literally drained away from Dad's face. I felt so sorry for my mother because I knew she probably would have loved to get onto the bed beside him and hold him, but it seemed impossible as the ICU was such a public place. All this time the people in the beds beside Dad's were watching and listening. I felt bad for them, too, because it was not a nice thing for anyone to have to see. During the last few minutes, the nurses continued to work away around us, wheeling patients in and out, and the contrast between those patients and Dad seemed very stark.

Dad's heartbeat got slower and slower and then the doctor came over and listened to his heart with a stethoscope and said he was gone. My tough, funny, capable, strong, dependable, full-of-life Dad, was gone for ever. I still can't believe that I'll never see him again.

The doctor then asked us to leave so that they could do whatever it is they do when people die. We asked if he could be put into a private room at this stage so that Mum could say her very last goodbyes and because my Dad's sister was on her way and she would like to see him, too. The staff asked us to wait for about half an hour and then came and took us to a room in the basement, to where they had brought Dad. My niece and Daniel thought they would go into the room first, just to make sure everything was OK, and I was so pleased that they did because it was difficult to see Dad lying on a trolley, wrapped in a sheet: all you could see was his face, which was pure white and waxy-looking. His head was hanging off the end of the trolley, so my niece, Aideen, got a pillow and propped his head up a bit. It was still a horrible way to see him and he didn't look at all like himself. Dad had to have an autopsy because of the way he died, so two orderlies had to stand beside the trolley waiting to take him away. That was the last time I saw my wonderful father.

Dad had an absolutely marvellous life. He lived it to the full and did everything he wanted to do. He left this earth exactly as he would have wanted to and for that I am very grateful. He always said he would die before he was eighty (he was seventy-eight) and he always wanted to go out, as he said, 'with a bang'! He did literally go with a bang and he knew nothing about it. No suffering and no realisation that he was leaving the world. Wouldn't we all wish for that? I can only sum up my dad by saying: 'He was some man for one man.'

My mother faced Dad's death with great dignity and has been coping well ever since. Everyone who has ever met her has described her as 'a lady', and this sums her up perfectly. I would consider her to be one of my best allies. She is a wonderful caring, gentle, giving person, never judgemental of other people. She would never allow us to gossip about other people's misfortunes when we were growing up: I remember that very clearly as a teenager and I always admired her for that. I could and do talk to Mum about everything in my life. She is very approachable and always gives good advice. She wanted all of us to enjoy life and to be happy.

As I have got older, I realize that I can't separate the 'mother' in Mum from the 'friend'. I don't want to hurt the mother so sometimes I have to keep things to myself that I really want the friend's advice on because I know that the 'mother' part of her would worry. I see that with my own children now. I want to know how they are getting on, but I don't want to hear all their problems because I would be upset that things weren't going right for them. All that would happen then is that I would bring myself down and that wouldn't help anyone. That is, unless I could do something about it!

You have to realize at some point in life that you need to solve or at least try to solve your own problems and not to expect others to sort everything for you. Sometimes, when my kids talk to me, they just want someone to listen to them. They don't need me to fix their problem, but just to listen and to understand. Mum is very good at that. If she thinks you're wrong about something, she will tell you straight out. I know lots of families where the children could do no wrong in their parents' eyes, but that was not the case with Mum or Dad. If you were out of order, they would very quickly let you know, even if it meant standing up for someone else above you. They would not fluff you up. I admire that. It's honest and straightforward.

Mum and Dad's relationship was typical of one formed in the 1950s, where the man did the earning and the wife did the rearing. Mum did everything and expected very little in return. She had great fun with Dad and there was never a dull moment in their lives. She always did what Dad wanted and never really questioned him. His clothes were always clean and his dinner was always ready. I think he was a very lucky man. Apart from being a very good wife/housewife, she was also very good-looking and still is to this day. She has a very good eye for style and for putting things together. Hmmm . . . maybe that's where my daughter Siobhan got it from. You would turn your head when Mum walked into a room. She has a very elegant way about her. I think my Dad was very proud to have her on his arm and in his life. He was always aware of what a gem he had and often said so.

It's very strange to think that my dad had such a big influence on me, yet it's my mother who was the constant in my life and was always there. I owe her so much. She was tough when she had to be, but always in a kind way. I know that she had hard times while we were growing up, as many people did, but she never let us see that. It's funny to realize that as I sit here writing about her, I find the words harder to find than when I talk about Dad. She is everything that Dad wasn't. I'm very lucky that I had that balance in my life. I love her to bits and I just cannot imagine my life without her.

Like many daughters, I suppose I take her for granted at times and it's only since Dad died that I realize that she won't be around for ever, so I try to spoil Mum a bit. When I go away travelling with Daniel, I always think of her and what she would like. When I see certain clothes, I say to myself, 'That's definitely the kind of thing Mum would wear', and I'll buy it for her. It gives me a lot of pleasure because I know that she will be happy with it. Sometimes she'll give out to me for spending money on her, but I tell her that it makes me feel good to see her enjoy something, especially things for the house. As I mentioned before, Dad had no real interest in doing up the house, but Mum loved it, so I buy her little nick-knacks that I think she would like. Dad would just think it was wasted money!

Mum is very easy to please and very undemanding. Any time I call her, she is delighted to hear from me and always thanks me for doing so. Even if I haven't called in a while, she never moans or gives out, she's just happy to hear from me. She understands that my life is very hectic at times and she never pressurizes me. She is always supportive of what I want to do in my life.

Mum and Dad were never in each other's pockets, which I think is a very healthy thing. They did lots together, but they also did things with their own friends. Now that Dad has gone, that's a very good thing because Mum is able to get on with the rest of her life. If we look at our lives as a book, we have the first few chapters, when we are growing up and single. Then we meet someone and they become part of our life story for the next however many chapters and then they leave our lives and we have the last few chapters on our own again. That's how I tried to explain it to Mum when we were talking about Dad's death. Yes, Dad was a major part of Mum's 'book' for fifty-eight years but, in the end, she will live the last few chapters by herself. Of course, this is sad in so many ways, but all of us are individuals with our own private thoughts and experiences of life. We never truly know someone in their entirety, much as we may think we do. There is always a part of us and our thoughts that no one else ever sees. That is life and, as you come into it, you also leave it: on your own.

Mum still has a few chapters left in her book and she will fill those chapters as fully as she can. Now is the time for her to look after herself for a change. That's hard to do when you have spent your whole life looking after other people as many, many mothers will know. I will do my best to make sure that my mum is content and happy in her final years. After all, it's the least I can do to repay her for the sacrifices she made for me. To sum my mum up, I would say, 'She is my hero'. And to sum my parents up, I wouldn't be the person I am today without them. None of us would be who we are without our parents. When I was younger, I always thought that they should be perfect and it disappointed me that they weren't, but it was only as I got older that I realized that none of us is perfect and all we can do is our best with the knowledge that we have at the time. My parents' love and support, and their flaws, made me who I am.

Chapter 4

LEARNING TO FLY

After I left school, I moved to Dublin to live with my parents. I got a job in a bakery, where I would make dough-nuts, fill cream cakes and pastries and serve at the counter. I enjoyed it, but I really wanted to have my freedom and while I lived at home, this was not going to happen. I wanted to spread my wings and go out into the big wide world, but I had to get some money together first. I don't think there was anything in particular that I wanted to do apart from singing and unless someone was going to walk up to me in the street and ask me to sing, that wasn't going to happen. A friend of mine in Dublin did ask if I would be the lead singer in his band and I think we did one gig, which was great, but that was it.

My boyfriend from Thurles had moved to London, so I decided that I wanted to go there. I desperately wanted to be with him, so I convinced my mum and dad to let me go, which they did, provided that I stayed with an aunt who was living in London at the time. After a few months, though, I wanted to spread my wings and have a bit more fun. A few of my friends from Thurles were staying in an apartment, which only had two bedrooms, but anyone from home was always welcome to stay, and so I moved in with them. I lived out of a suitcase and slept on the floor, but that didn't make any difference to me.

I had a fantastic time when I was there. A couple of the guys from Pyramid lived in the apartment and at night we would sit around in a circle and listen to music, play the guitar and sing. I relished the freedom and loved the chance to sing at any opportunity. I wasn't doing anything publicly, but that didn't matter. As long as I could sing, that was fine. At one stage, there must have been eight or nine people living in the apartment and I don't know how we all managed with one bathroom, but we did!

I was also hoping that my romance, which my boyfriend had finished shortly after he moved to London, would reignite, but that wasn't to be. After about eight months, I had to accept that he had met someone else and that I had been rejected. (I use that word deliberately as I will explain later – the feeling of rejection has been such a strong force for me in my life.) My world just fell apart. I was devastated because I had thought that he was the one for me. I was only eighteen years of age and I remember being very down and crying a lot. I suppose the rejection itself was the hardest part and feeling that I was unloved by someone I cared about so much because when I look back, it was all very innocent and would never have worked out. Really, I was only a child. However, even though I wasn't aware of it at the time, I suppose that was the first time that I had ever experienced rejection. It was a long time before I would realize why being rejected impacted on me so significantly.

About three months after that, myself and a couple of girlfriends decided to get an apartment on our own. We had very little money, so the choice was very limited. I remember the apartment very well – in fact, I don't think I'll ever forget it! As we had so little money, the only place we could afford was in Harlesden in north-west London and it was a sad affair to say the least! There were four of us and the apartment had only one bedroom. There was a single bed and a set of bunk-beds and the last girl to join us in the apartment had to rotate between the three beds every week, sleeping top to tail with each of us in turn. There was a small sitting room with a gas fire and off that, the smallest kitchenette you have ever seen. There was literally a cooker, sink and, believe it or not, a bath tub, which had a lid on it that was used as the work surface in the kitchen. I really don't know how landlords got away with it, but they did because there were so many people just like us, with very little money and low expectations, looking for some place to stay. At that stage, I was earning £19 a week working as a bought-ledger clerk at Ladbrokes head office in London and the rent on the apartment was £7 a week. The rest was used for food, transport, entertainment and whatever else I needed.

Even though the apartment was appalling, we had great times and I have fond memories of when we lived there. I can remember having a bath and being able to stir the pot on the cooker at the same time! Because we had very little money, we just sat in and played cassettes most nights, but I loved the freedom. I loved the fact that I could do anything I wanted whenever I wanted. That's a very simple thing, but when you have been restricted all your life, it's amazing when those restrictions are lifted. I didn't have to answer to anyone and that suited me fine. It wasn't that I was up to anything bad, far from it, it was just that for the first time in my life it was *my* choice to do as I wished with my life.

It was 1978. Life was simple and mainly consisted of going to work every day and staying in at night with friends. I didn't really drink much or go to pubs because I just didn't have the money to do that, but I never got into the Irish scene in London, even though I started out in Cricklewood with my aunt. I made friends at work and, regardless of what nationality they were, they became my social life. One girl I worked with at Ladbrokes was called Mary and her parents were originally from Ireland, even though Mary and her brother and sisters had all been born in London. She lived with her mum and dad and would often ask me around for dinner. As I didn't have much money or interest in cooking at that time, I loved to go. Her mother, also called Mary, did a great dinner of bacon and cabbage with boiled potatoes: it was like going home. They had the Sacred Heart picture with the eternal flame underneath in the living room and they played Irish music and embraced everything Irish. Their home was a little slice of Ireland, and this was typical of many Irish people in London. I find that the Irish abroad are much more 'Irish' than the Irish at home, if you know what I mean. I think that's what happens when we leave our own place – we almost go overboard trying never to forget where we came from. I like that, but I also like to mix with my new surroundings. I think it's important to embrace a different culture while always remembering and respecting your own.

I made some good friends in London and, even though our lives have gone in different directions, I still see Mary and keep in contact with her to this day. Or should I say, she keeps in contact with me. I have to admit that I am useless when it comes to staying in touch with people. That is a bad fault, which I must work on. I am godmother to one of her children and it's lovely to see all the twists and turns that life has taken in the thirty-six years I have known her.

When I was nineteen years old, I moved into a house with another girl I had met at work. Denise lived with her brother and I was fascinated with her because she was so sophisticated; I had never met anyone like her before. Even though I was almost a grown woman, I didn't wear make-up or own a handbag or care what I wore, which always involved jeans! I hardly ever wore a dress. It was just too uncomfortable and it usually meant you had to wear tights.

Ugh! I was a real tomboy. Denise, on the other hand, was the complete opposite. She was about seven years older than me and very English in an almost Cockney kind of way. She would put her hair in curlers every single day. I thought that was pure torture and couldn't understand why anyone would want to do that. Then she would bring all her make-up into the sitting room and begin to apply it in a very methodical way. When she was finished and had removed all the curlers, she was stunning. She was very good-looking with beautiful long shiny jet-black hair, big brown eyes and the most captivating smile, with beautiful white teeth and voluptuous lips. That was it! I wanted to be like her.

Thanks to Denise, it suddenly dawned on me that I was a woman and that I should try to look and behave like one. I bought my first handbag and felt like a fish out of water using it, but I persevered. I bought make-up and had my hair permed. I thought I was gorgeous, but to tell you the truth, I was a sight. I used to wear blue eye shadow all over my eyelids and that was the only colour I possessed.

I am definitely one of those people who improves with age, like a good wine. I was very, very plain then, with awful hair that I could do nothing with. We did have hair dryers, but we didn't have all the other gadgets that young people have now: straighteners, fake tan, gels, mousses, waxing, Botox, padded bras that push you up and pull you in and make you look three sizes bigger and all the other wonderful stuff that we have to enhance ourselves these days. I mean, I've even seen padded knickers that make your bum look more shapely – what chance did we have at all in the Seventies?

Apart from being beautiful, Denise could flirt for England. She was a real natural. If a man looked in her direction, she would confidently smile back at him and bat her eyelids in a very flattering way. If a man looked in my direction, I would turn around and look behind me to see if there was someone else there. I could never believe that he would actually be looking at me! I had no confidence whatsoever. I had to know a person well before anything would happen romantically because I never recognized the signs that someone was flirting with me. I think you need confidence to flirt and, at that time, I certainly didn't have confidence.

I really admired Denise and I learned a lot from her. Her brother, who was about nine years older than me and divorced, was also very English and I loved his accent. I thought he was so sophisticated and worldly. He had a moustache and I thought that he was a real man, as opposed to the boys whom I had dated before. He was really nice to me and I enjoyed his company. We became a couple and once again, thanks to the new man in my life, I thought it was sorted.

I was twenty when he asked me to marry him and I thought, not, 'Do I love him?' but, 'Finally someone wants me'. I said 'yes'. We bought an apartment together and moved in and I was so happy. Someone loved me and wanted to spend the rest of his life with me. But after about a year, I thought that something wasn't quite right. It wasn't something I could put my finger on, but I just knew that I wasn't happy in the relationship. Some people might call it gut instinct or intuition, in which I am a great believer. I suppose I didn't believe that it was possible for someone to love me. I couldn't believe that I could be so lucky, so I kept testing his love for me. If I pushed him away from me, would he come back? I was afraid I was going to lose him and that terrified me, so I finished with him to see if he would miss me so much that he would travel to the ends of the earth and do anything to get me back. Then I would know for sure that he really did love me.

The reality is, at the time I couldn't love myself, so it was unlikely that anyone else was going to love me, no matter what I did. If he had pursued me, I probably would have tested him in some other way, as I would never believe that I could be loved. I left London and moved back to Ireland, hoping he would ask me to come back. As it turned out, my plan backfired: he didn't want me back and that was the end of that relationship.

Once again, I fell apart. The rejection was unbearable. I went back to London again, hoping that I could win him back, but he had moved on and met someone else. I was very depressed for a long time and I thought that I would be better off out of this world. I felt I couldn't handle any more pain. I never did anything about these suicidal thoughts because I didn't have the guts, but the thoughts were there. I got no joy from anything. It was as if I was dead inside and I just felt like a burden to everyone. I didn't realize that I was depressed. I just thought that this was what happened when someone left you. I thought everyone felt and behaved the same way. I spent most of my time in bed or watching television and it was my good friends at the time who fed me and put up with me and kept me going. I was only twenty-one, but it was my first real experience of depression and it took me almost a year to get over that break-up.

A pattern was definitely emerging, but I didn't see it at the time. I desperately wanted to settle down with someone, but I sabotaged it every time. I couldn't stop myself. It was a negative cycle that I couldn't break. I don't even know if I was aware of it at the time. It was just a case of, 'Poor me. Nobody loves me. What's wrong with me?'

Somehow, I pulled myself out of my depression. I managed to find a new job after a few months and life once again started to settle down. I went to work at Wembley Stadium Conference Centre and Arena. That was a really great place to work. I was involved in lots of interesting events and concerts, with artists such as Michael Jackson, David Bowie, Tina Turner, the original Live Aid concert, the Benson & Hedges Masters snooker tournament, as well as major football matches. I was a cashier at the time and when the large concerts were on, we would have to get a lot of casual staff, as they were called, to cover all the work. We would have to count all the money from the bars and stands all around the stadium during the events. At the end of the day, we would have trays and trays of notes to count and sometimes it was impossible to get the money to balance because the notes would be soaking wet and covered in beer: you were literally peeling them apart to count them. We had to balance the books to within £5 or we would have to start all over again. I am talking about thousands of wet pounds in cash here! In spite of that, I have to say that I really enjoyed it. I got to get out and about during the events and it gave me a real sense of satisfaction when we did balance the books after a long day.

I remember about a year later, after I had moved to Glasgow to work, one of my ex-colleagues at the stadium asked if I wanted to work on the Michael Jackson concert, as she needed extra staff. I was going out with Raymond at the time, whom I would later marry, and we decided that we would go to London for the weekend so he could do casual work as well. As he was a banqueting manager, they said they would find something for him to do. I was pleased that Raymond would get to see where and who I worked with and what was involved.

I was up in the cash office, organizing floats to send to the bars, when Raymond came in and told me that they had a wee job for him to do. As it turned out, Princess Diana was attending the concert and she was in the royal box. Management needed someone with experience to wait on them and who do you think got the job? None other than the bold Raymond. I was so jealous. There was me showing him what Wembley was like and how important my job was and he ended up in the royal box with Princess Diana and Michael Jackson!

*

Before Raymond came into my life, I met a gorgeous guy while working in Wembley and fell head over heels again. Now, this guy was a looker. Tall, dark and very handsome, and guess what? He liked me! Back on the rollercoaster that was my love life, I was on the up again. I couldn't believe my luck. The only down side was that he had already made plans to travel to Hong Kong to work there for a year, so I knew that it would not be straightforward.

After about eight months, he made his final travel plans and was heading off. He was stopping in Thailand for a two-week holiday on the way and suggested that I go with him for that break. I was twenty-three at this time and I was delighted with myself as we headed off to Thailand. I was absolutely sure that he would work in Hong Kong for a few months to a year and that he would come back and settle down with me.

We had the most wonderful time in Thailand. The people there are beautiful; so friendly. We travelled to pretty remote places and the locals kept coming up and asking me to have my picture taken with them because my skin was so white in comparison to theirs. We went to the island of Koh Samui and rented a shack on the beach for a few days. It was like heaven on earth. I know that there is an airport and that there are lots of hotels on the island nowadays, but in 1983, it was very different. The shack was literally a few feet from the water's edge. There were coconut trees all around it and you could just pick up a fallen coconut from the beach and eat it. The shack was pretty rough and ready, just big enough for a bed and a toilet area. The bed was a mattress on a plinth and the toilet was a hole in the ground; the shower consisted of a hose sticking out of the wall. The shacks were owned by local families and we ate our breakfast and dinner with them. Every night after dinner, they would offer us a cookie from a cookie jar, which we would happily take as we strolled back down the moonlit beach. We soon discovered that they were hash cookies. I have to say that the walk back down the beach to the shack each night was a very pleasant one because of those cookies!

The island was idyllic and the sand was like white flour. The sea was a clear blue and the water was always welcoming. You could spend hours in it and never feel cold. I remember that for the first couple of days we were there, I thought I would die of boredom, but then I really started to relax as I had never done before. We were up each morning at about six o'clock and in bed each night by seven o'clock. All we did during the day was walk and read and swim. At the end of the two weeks, it was time for me to go home. The parting was very emotional on both our parts and I felt sure that we would be together again. I visited him once for a holiday in Hong Kong and we had a wonderful time.

While we were apart that year, letters were very frequently exchanged. I thought about him constantly, but after about six months, the letters became less frequent. He was away about a year altogether when I received a 'Dear John' letter. The 'it's not you, it's me' kind of thing. He told me that he was not coming back from Hong Kong as he had a great job and a new life there. I couldn't understand it. I felt that he was only having doubts because he hadn't seen me for a while and I was sure that if he did spend some time with me, we would be OK. So I decided that even though I didn't have much money, I would scrape together what I had and I would get on a plane and go out there and see him. It couldn't end with a letter.

So, off I went on my own to Hong Kong. Because the ticket was the lowest fare I could get, I had to go all over the place to get there, with ridiculous stop-overs in between of anything between two and six hours, but I'm like a terrier when I get an idea in my head and nothing will stop me, no matter how much discomfort I put myself through. I think all together it took two days for me to get to Hong Kong. My boyfriend picked me up at the airport, but I could see straight away that there was a distance in his eyes. I tried desperately to convince him that he still loved me and that we could make a go of it, but I got nowhere. I think he had met someone else. So, after only three days, I got back on the plane and cried all the way home. Now came the down of the roller coaster, with more heartbreak and loneliness.

I worked and existed for the next few months, once again in that dark, lonely place in my head. And then, after a while, one of my bosses was moving to Scotland and asked me if I was interested in a job there. I was to be employed as a conference and banqueting co-ordinator at the Hospitality Inn (as it was known at the time) on Sauchiehall Street in Glasgow. As nothing special, or should I say nobody special, was happening in my life at that time, I thought it would be a good opportunity to move away from all that London reminded me of. And so, I moved to Glasgow and stayed with my boss and his partner until I found a small bedsit of my own, in a house with about six other bedsits and a kitchen that we all shared. There was no communal sitting room, so unless we were cooking, we were in our respective rooms. I made my little place as comfortable as possible and bought little bits and pieces to brighten up the place. I had learned to do that from my mum. I worked hard and didn't mind doing so because I knew nobody in Glasgow at the time, so I wasn't socialising.

I loved the job and volunteered for everything going. It was an office job and would finish at around six p.m., but if there was an event going on in the hotel, I would stay and do whatever needed to be done. It was a great learning curve because I got to be involved in events from the very beginning to the very end. It was a very large hotel with banqueting facilities for one thousand people and it had sixteen private function rooms altogether. Usually a co-ordinator would meet a client initially and discuss their requirements, show them a suitable function room and take down every detail of the event to pass onto the conference and banqueting manager. That would be the extent of a co-ordinator's role, but I wanted to be involved in the whole process. It meant that I worked long hours for no extra pay, but it was well worth it in the end because of the valuable experience I gained during that time.

I didn't set out to get involved in hotel management, but that is what I ended up doing and if you're going to do something, you may as well give it your best shot. I lived alone in a bedsit, so I was happy to be out and doing something worthwhile rather then sitting at home alone and I liked the fact that I was dealing with different people every day.

The assistant conference and banqueting manager was called Raymond and he was a very charming and funny guy. He paid me loads of attention and gave me lots of compliments, which I really liked. Who wouldn't? I was living in a bedsit on my own and it was pretty lonely when I wasn't at work. He had a nice car and was very particular about how he dressed. He was very confident, which I always liked in a man. I was attracted to him, but at that stage, he was very casually seeing someone else at the hotel. He then decided to buy an apartment in Glasgow and needed someone to share to help pay the mortgage. Of course, I was more than happy to oblige because it gave me a better standard of living for the same money and I liked him. I subsequently moved in as his lodger. After a few weeks, we went to a friend's house for dinner and at the end of the night, we ended up kissing. Oh no! Here we go again! I did nothing by half measures and I was never a casual dater. It was all or nothing with me. So now, I was living with the guy I was dating, which was a bit backwards. It was all going very fast and I suppose I was happy with that because a relationship was all I'd ever wanted.

I was on cloud nine and thought that, this time, I'd found 'the one'. On reflection, there were a few things which should have made me cautious, but it wasn't in my nature. I remember being in bed one morning around Easter time and he brought me in an Easter egg as he left for work. I thought it was so thoughtful because no one had ever done anything like that for me before, but then, later that day, I discovered another Easter egg in the apartment and when I asked him about it, he told me it was for the other girl that he had been seeing!

I should have realized then that he was a player, but I thought I could 'change him'. I know now that you can never change anyone. You can only change yourself and then maybe they will change their behaviour towards you. But I had yet to learn that lesson, and so I brushed it off and told him he was a cheeky bugger and at that point he said that our relationship would be exclusive. Everything seemed perfect and I was on the up again.

Isn't it amazing that everything in my life revolved around men? They were the ones who made me happy or sad. It was totally in their control. How wrong I was. I have learned over the years and many heartbreaks, that while we might not have control over what happens to us, all of us have control over what we think and how we react. We just have to take that control and use it. I spent so many years blaming other people for my unhappiness when, in fact, I was responsible for my own happiness in life.

We had only been dating for about three months when Raymond asked me to marry him. It was a strange proposal because it was almost as if it were a business agreement. He pointed out that we got on well together and that we were a good team and that we should look at marriage practically rather than romantically. That seemed fine to me at the time because I had been out with four other guys whom I thought I could have married, so maybe all this romantic stuff was all bull. Don't get me wrong, I loved him and he was very romantic, but I thought that being practical as well wasn't such a bad thing. He was good marriage material and I thought he would be a good provider for his family. So we got engaged in May and we were married in September of the same year. Talk about a whirlwind romance. I married Raymond in 1986 in a small village outside Glasgow called Uddingston. I was on top of the world and thought that I had finally met the man with whom I would spend the rest of my life.

Chapter 5

CRASHING TO EARTH

When I look back on it now, I have no idea why Raymond decided to marry me at all. It was something I never found out or could get him to explain. However, I want to talk about that marriage in this chapter in full because I need to share what I experienced so that you will better understand how I got to where I am today. Although there are some 'not very nice truths' here, this is not about blaming anyone. We both did the best we could at the time. I have learned a lot since then and I'm sure Raymond has, too. Nowadays, we have a very amicable relationship and Daniel and I have met Raymond and his wife Teresa on a few occasions.

I called Raymond to tell him that I was writing this

book and that I wanted to be very honest about the breakdown of the marriage. He was fine with it and appreciated the fact that I had mentioned it to him. As Raymond rightly said to me, this is *my* perception of what happened. I'm sure his would be very different, but all I can do is tell you how I saw it. As they say, 'Perception is reality to those perceiving'. I have no bad feelings for Raymond and I certainly would never wish him any harm because, at the end of the day, he is the father of my children and I can never change that.

When we were planning our wedding, I realized that there was no point in me going back to have the ceremony in my home town of Thurles because Mum and Dad didn't live there any more, or any of my family. We decided to stay in Scotland and we found a lovely, very small, church, which only seated about one hundred people. I was so happy on that day and I didn't feel a bit nervous. I thought I was the luckiest girl in the world. Raymond was tall, handsome, confident, funny and knew an awful lot about an awful lot. And what's more, he wanted to marry me. My family were happy because they had met Raymond and they thought that he was a decent guy. They felt that he was very sensible and would look after me well.

We had the whole works as far as a white wedding was concerned. The dress was made of white lace, very fitted, with a fishtail bottom to it. It had long sleeves, all puffed at the top, which was the fashion at the time. I got it in a bridal shop in Glasgow and it cost me about £450. It had been in the shop for some time and I bought it off the rack, probably a 'sale' rack, knowing me! Anyway, it was not as white as it should have been, so I decided to wash it in the bath. I ran some tepid water, put in a little washing powder and laid the dress on top. I didn't want to be rough with it or handle it too much so I took my shoes and socks off, got into the bath and just walked up and down on the dress as the water turned a very dirty colour. It certainly needed that wash. I then hung it up over the bath and let it drip dry. The next day it looked perfect! Job well done and lots of money saved. 'Practical' is my middle name. My veil was very short and it was attached to a headband of pearls.

I suppose we all look back at our wedding photos and think we looked awful or 'a sight', as they say in Donegal, but I really did – in all seriousness, I was lovely at the time, but I can't help thinking that I looked so young and naïve.

As I walked down the aisle that day, I felt so happy and

that I'd finally accomplished what I had always wanted. Just to belong and be loved. All I needed now was a baby and then I would be fulfilled, or so I thought.

Sure enough, after our honeymoon, we went back to our apartment (it was 'ours' now that we were married!) and I was on cloud nine when after six months, I found out I was pregnant with my first child. I cannot even put into words how that made me feel. I had always had it in my head that I would die young and never have the chance to have children, but I was proven wrong. For the first time in my life, I felt like a real grown-up. I was going to be a mammy.

I did everything right and read up on everything to make sure that I was as prepared as I could be before the birth. Raymond was really good and was as excited as I was. Well, I think he was anyway. To be honest, I don't know what he really was thinking the whole time we were together. I thought I did and he certainly gave me the impression that he was happy, but when what you think and believe is completely turned upside down, you start to question everything. I asked Raymond so many times about how he felt or if he was happy and he always said yes. He obviously found it hard to be honest and open with me. Even to this day I have no idea why he did what he did or what it was in our marriage that made it impossible for him to work through. I guess that's his story to tell. I can only say what I saw, heard and felt was the case.

I put on a lot of weight during my first pregnancy. I was eight stone when I got married and I went up to thirteen stone when I was nine months' pregnant. I was huge everywhere. My arms, neck, thighs and bum were massive. Talk about stretch marks! I would say they were more stretch tears and I had them all over my stomach and thighs. My body never was the same again. I don't know why I put on so much weight, but I did. I see some young girls now having babies and if you were walking behind them, you wouldn't know they were pregnant. All they have is a baby belly. Lucky them. Anyway, apart from my weight gain, everything went very smoothly during the pregnancy and I had no problems whatsoever. I looked forward to motherhood and I prepared for it. I used to play classical music to the baby by putting headphones on my stomach and we both believed that talking to it was very important. I kept telling the baby that it was due to arrive on 1 December and that we were ready and waiting. I would say how much we were looking forward to meeting him or her. (We didn't know the sex of the baby and I didn't want to know. In those days, they only told you if there was a problem and you only got a photo of the scan if there was a problem with the baby, so none of that for us.) We bought flash cards to teach the baby to read and to learn words to make sure we would raise a really intelligent person.

While I was pregnant, Raymond and I decorated the spare room as a nursery and as I was getting close to the end of the nine months, I used to go into it and sit on my rocking chair and look at all the lovely baby clothes, the cot with the bumper and the mobile in it and the pushchair and pram. The walls were decorated with bunny rabbits and Noddy pictures. I reflected on how lucky I was to have everything that I had. There I was, sitting with my baby in my tummy, eager for it to arrive, knowing that everything was ready and waiting. I was happy because I had a husband who was a good provider, good around the house and was excited at the prospect of his first child's arrival. What more could anyone ask for in life? I had it cracked.

Of course, things would turn out differently, but at the time, all I could see was my happy future stretching ahead of me. It might seem odd now, but I remember feeling relieved that I wouldn't be alone. I never wanted to be a lone parent and I didn't have to be now, I thought. I had wondered in the past what I might do if I got pregnant accidentally: would I have a baby on my own? I just felt that I wouldn't be able to manage. As it happens, I certainly wouldn't have managed! I was too insecure and dependent to have brought another person into the world by myself. I know differently now and it just goes to show you that there are no guarantees in life. I waited for what I thought was the right person to have a family with, but ended up alone anyway.

I went into labour on 30 November 1987 and my daughter, Siobhán, was born on 1 December, her due date. I was convinced that she arrived because I had been telling her when she was due to arrive. My labour was very long, about thirty hours and at the end of it, I had to have a Caesarean section. She was making no headway at all and I was stuck at nine centimetres – you need to be ten before you can push – for seven hours. They decided that we were both too tired, so the section was carried out and I was so glad because I was wrecked.

When she was born, Siobhán had the most amazing presence, which I really didn't expect. Her eyes were wide open, her face was smooth and relaxed and she just looked around the room, as if she was taking it all in and knew exactly what was happening: 'Wow, I'm here. So this is what the world looks like'. When I got the chance to be with her a few hours after she was born, I fell absolutely and utterly in love with her. I thought she was *the* most beautiful baby that had ever been born. Of course, we all think that about our babies and rightly so. That's nature doing its job.

I laid her on the hospital bed and I examined every little bit of her. I was in absolute awe of her. She was perfect in every way and I couldn't get over the size of her little toes and nails and fingers. I loved her smell and I loved kissing her neck between her ear and her shoulder. And she was all mine. I made her. I grew her all by myself.

Of course, she was Raymond's baby, too, but I didn't think it was possible for him to have that bond that a mother and baby have. I had known her for the previous nine months. I had felt her move and kick. He was just meeting her now. I looked at Raymond to see if he felt the same amazement at witnessing his first baby arrive in the world and he was crying. This made me so happy because I knew something in him had been awakened. I don't think he realized that he was going to feel as he did. He told me years after we had separated that he only really started to love me after Siobhán was born.

Of course, I was every bit the overprotective mum. I

remember when they came to do the neonatal heel-prick test, the one that they do on all newborns, I genuinely thought that my baby was 'special' and that she needed to be treated gently, not just like all the other babies. She was an angel on earth and should be treated as such. Instead, they stuck the needle into her heel and squeezed until they got a drop of blood. She roared. And then I roared!! I thought they were torturing her. How could they do that to my poor new baby? She was only in the world one day and already someone was causing her pain. I'm sure most mothers feel the same, but at the time, I thought I was the only one.

I had to stay in hospital for seven days as I had had a C-section and I can tell you, I got very little sleep. I would have been far better off at home, where I could have slept in my own bed whenever I needed to. I was ridiculously happy for about four days and on the fifth, I vividly remember walking down the corridor to the bathroom. I sat on the toilet with a big smile on my face and about two minutes later, I was howling my eyes out. The realisation had just hit me: Oh, my God, I thought, I am this child's mother and she depends totally on me for everything. How can I possibly know what to do. What if I let her fall or she chokes on something and I panic, or I lose her somewhere and on and on and on ... I was terrified. My hormones were all over the place and I now think that I was experiencing the first signs of post-natal depression.

On the seventh day, I left hospital and we went home with our new daughter. We were now a family. As I started my new life with a baby, I genuinely thought that I would never have a hot cup of tea or meal again as long as I lived! I couldn't believe how much of my time she took up. Maybe it was just because she was constantly on my mind as she was my first, but babies seem to take up every moment. I kept waiting for her to wake up and if she made a sound when she was asleep, I was straight into the bedroom to see if she was OK.

I can vividly remember the first time I went out with her in the pram for a walk. We lived near the centre of Glasgow at the time, so I decided to go to the shops. After about an hour, Siobhán started to cry and I didn't know what to do. I ran the whole way home so that I could take her out of the pram to see what was wrong with her. I could probably have done that in town, but it was all so overwhelming at the time.

Those first few months were very tough and Siobhán was a very demanding baby. She had a reflux problem for the first two months and she would promptly throw up her bottle as soon as she was finished it. Now, I am not talking about a bit of milk down her front: I am talking projectile vomiting. I would give her a bottle, but as soon as I sat her up to burp her, practically the whole bottle of milk would shoot across the floor out of her mouth. We would be back to square one because she would be hungry again and I would need to give her another feed! After about two months, the carpet was full of white stain marks about five feet in length.

During this time, Raymond's mother, Margaret, was a tower of strength to me. She took Siobhán the odd day so that I could catch up on my sleep, which I so desperately needed and still do to this day. I need about ten hours' sleep each night to function normally. If I miss a couple of nights that's OK, but no longer than that. At that time, I just wasn't getting enough sleep. A crying baby can really push you to the edge when you are exhausted, but I was not only exhausted, I was also very depressed.

I remember one time Siobhán was crying so much that I wanted to shake her. I realized that the way I felt wasn't right and I immediately held her in my arms and asked her for forgiveness. I was disgusted with myself. It never occurred to me that I had depression. I just presumed that this was what it was like for everyone and I just had to get on with it. I think it is so important for young mothers to know that post-natal depression is a very common thing and that they should not be afraid to ask for help if they feel they need it. It is not a sign of weakness, but of strength. It takes a strong person to admit that she needs help and an even stronger person to actually ask for it. You owe it to your baby and to yourself.

As I said, my mother-in-law was wonderful in that way. She was a great help to me as I didn't have my own mother around at that time. Mum and Dad were still living in Dublin then, but I would never have dreamed of calling them up to say that I couldn't cope. They had their own lives to be getting on with and I am not a very good person at asking for, or accepting, help. I don't know why that is. I suppose I was brought up with the attitude that I had to just 'get on with it and stop moaning' and that's what I thought I had to do.

As the months passed, though, Siobhán settled and started to sleep at night, which made life a lot easier. Raymond was a great dad and he involved himself with looking after Siobhán whenever he could. Things seemed finally to be settling down. Then, about two years after Siobhán was born, I became pregnant again and I was delighted with myself, but when I was about twelve weeks along, I went for a scan and they couldn't find a heartbeat. I had miscarried. I was admitted to hospital, where they carried out a dilation and curettage, or D&C, as it's more commonly known, to remove the foetus from the uterus in case of infection. I was very upset and disappointed, but I figured that it was nature's way of telling me that something was wrong, so I accepted it, even though I was so sad about it.

Raymond didn't really understand how I felt, or at least, it seemed that way to me. He seemed to find it difficult to address his emotions and tended to compartmentalize them. He had the ability to put parts of his life into a box and to not let one part impact on another or the people in it. This, of course, is just my view, but my view is all I can tell you about. As I mentioned earlier, I do not want to talk about Raymond in a negative way, even though there were things that he did at the time that were very hurtful to me.

Nonetheless, we decided to try for another baby. Raymond was the youngest of four and all of his siblings had had girls. There was not one boy to carry on the family name. Raymond read all sorts of things about how you could increase your chances of conceiving a boy and he tried a few of them, such as diet – eating a lot of fish and salty foods – wearing boxer shorts instead of briefs and lots of other things. There's lots of research on the Internet these days about it. Anyway, about six months later, I was pregnant again and we were really hoping for a boy, but very doubtful that it could happen. Again, I had a very healthy pregnancy, with no trouble at all. Because I'd had such a tough time with Siobhan's birth, I had an X-ray taken and it was discovered that some bone around my cervix was an unusual shape, which made it almost impossible for me to give birth naturally. So it was decided that I would have an elective Caesarean section. That was great because I knew when the big day would be and I was able to plan everything beforehand. The other plus is that I would be taken in two weeks before my due date, so that I would not go into labour myself. When you're pregnant and you're given a due date, that's the only date you have in your mind. You really don't think past that date, so when you do go over, it must be a real pain. Luckily, I never experienced that!

I was fully expecting a second daughter and then, after the operation, it was announced that it was a boy. I couldn't believe it! A boy. Now I had the perfect family. A daughter and a son. There wasn't any other kind, so I had it all. We called him Michael and we were both very proud and surprised.

His face was all screwed up when he came out and he was crying and struggling – totally different to Siobhán, who had been so serene. I was so happy to have my boy. I kept saying to the nurses and anyone who would listen, 'It's a boy. It's a boy. It's a boy'. I was also delighted because I experienced all the loving emotions with Michael that I had felt with Siobhán. When I was pregnant with Michael, I was afraid that I couldn't possibly love another child as much as I loved his sister. I loved her so deeply and absolutely and I really didn't think it was possible to be able to love two people like that. What if I didn't bond with Michael, I had wondered to myself. However, I have since realized that there's plenty of love to go around.

I also realize that the love you have for your child is so different to the love you have for a partner. Totally different, and I was just about to discover that with Michael. I needn't have worried at all. I fell in love with him as quickly and as deeply as I had with Siobhán.

Being a parent is amazing and a feeling that cannot be put into words, but only experienced. I don't think any of us really realize what our parents go through until we have children of our own. I ended up with a much greater respect for my mother in particular, when I became a mother myself. I really didn't give it a second thought before that. Times were so different when my mother was having me and my siblings. She was very ill when her first child, my brother Michael, was born. She developed pre-eclampsia and almost died, but as was so often the way at the time, nobody explained what was happening or what to expect and she never once questioned or complained about anything. She believed that she just had to do as she was told. She told me that she was very frightened. When she went on to have my sister, Josephine, she was understandably scared, but that fear was dismissed by the hospital staff – in those days, you simply did what you were told. Apparently, my birth was the best and easiest – need I say more!

Raymond and I had moved to Edinburgh by this stage, as he had been given the opportunity to set up and run a restaurant there. He had always wanted to be his own boss, so this was a step towards that. However, it meant working all the hours under the sun. He had a day off while we were still in hospital, but he couldn't visit us because he had stuff to do for the restaurant. I really admired him for his work ethic, even if we had no visit that day.

When I got out of hospital, we picked Siobhán up from Margaret and Alistair, Raymond's parents, and headed home with our two beautiful children. Raymond said that he was going out to 'wet the baby's head' with a few friends and that he wouldn't be late as he was taking the car, so he wouldn't be drinking. I was happy enough and settled Siobhán and my newborn down for the evening. As Michael was only seven days old, he needed feeding every four hours or so, so I was up during the night to see to him. The hours passed by and there was no sign of Raymond. One a.m. passed, then two a.m., three, four, five, six a.m., and still nothing. I was at my wits' end. He had said that he wouldn't be late and as it was my first night home with a toddler and a newborn after having a C-section, I was sure he would be home if he could. With no plausible explanation, my imagination started to run wild. I was sure he'd had an accident and was lying in a ditch somewhere. By eleven o'clock the next morning, I was hysterical. I called his parents in an awful state, crying and sobbing down the phone. They came to the house and tried to calm me while they made phone calls to a few of Raymond's friends to see if anyone had seen him. No one had.

At about two p.m., he walked in the front door with some excuse that he had fallen asleep on a friend's sofa and hadn't woken up. I slapped him hard and then threw my arms around him to hold him tight because I was so relieved that he was home. Thank God he isn't dead, was all I could think.

It wasn't until Michael was six months old that I found out that Raymond was having an affair and had been since before Michael was born. The day he had missed while I was in hospital and the night he didn't come home, he'd spent at her house, but all that was to hit me further down the line. At the time, I was completely unaware of it.

We moved house when Michael was only three weeks old and, as we had been living on the outskirts of Edinburgh, I was happy to be moving into the centre of the city. I remember that the apartment cost £102,000, which seemed like a lot of money in 1990, and I couldn't believe that we could actually afford a mortgage of that size. I was on maternity leave, but Raymond was doing pretty well financially at the restaurant. He was always bright and clever in coming up with ways to make money. It was a garden apartment in a big three-storey old house. The apartment was beautiful and I felt like a queen. The only problem was that Raymond was working such long hours at the restaurant and I was alone and, once again, experiencing post-natal depression. I still didn't realize that that's what it was. As the depression set in, I started to feel very isolated in the apartment. Even though we had a garden, which was a lovely space to have in the city, I still felt closed in because we were on the lower-ground floor, below street level. I used to feel like a rabbit coming out of its warren each time I came out to go to the shops.

Apart from that, something just didn't feel right between Raymond and myself. My instinct has always been very strong and usually it's right. I just knew that Raymond was behaving differently towards me. He seemed a little distracted and distant with me, but I had absolutely no reason to feel that something was going on. It was just pure instinct.

I started asking him if he was OK, if he was happy with me, even if he was having an affair. I wanted to know if he still loved me, but every time he would reassure me that everything was fine. I remember one time, he said that he loved his life with me and the children and that he couldn't understand why I was so doubtful of him. I started to doubt myself at this stage and wondered what was wrong with me. Why could I not just believe what he said? But my gut told me something different. I was fighting with my instincts constantly and the result was that I was feeling more and more depressed each day.

Also, because I was alone most of the time, I found it

hard to cope with the children, particularly Siobhán, as she was at the age when she needed attention and I just couldn't manage. One day in particular she was in bad form and she kept pulling at me and crying and I felt as though I was the child all of a sudden; as if I was the one who needed attention. Michael was six months old at this stage so he was easier to handle because all he did was sleep and eat. I was at my wits' end, so I went into the toilet with Michael in my arms and I called social services because I knew that I needed help. Siobhán was knocking on the door and asking me to come out, God love her.

When I think of it now, it makes me want to cry. I wish I could have both my children back at that age again now, while I am feeling good, so that I could smother them with kisses and cuddles. (It's a bit awkward when they're twenty-four and twenty-six!) I explained that I just needed a break and they organized for Siobhán to go to a child-minder on Monday to Friday from nine until five, to give me some quiet time. Perhaps you're wondering why I didn't ask Raymond's parents to help more. I think it's because I am a pretty proud person and I felt that they had done so much already when Siobhán was born. I didn't want them to think that I was a bad mother or that I couldn't cope. I was afraid that they would think that

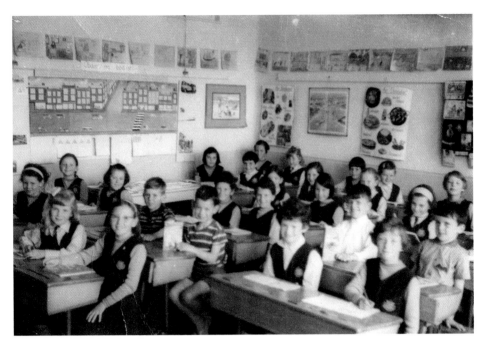

Presentation Convent Primary School, Thurles, County Tipperary, 1968. That's me in the front on the right.

My debs ball in Thurles, 1978. I'm the one in the front on the left – bad curl day!

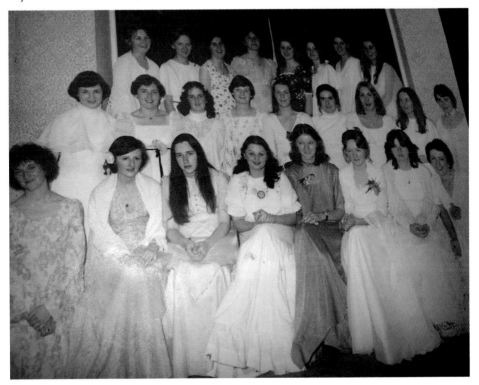

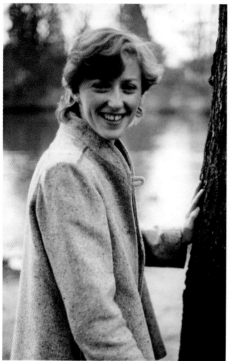

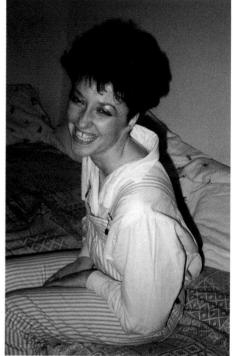

A photo taken when I was about 20 and living in London.

In my Glasgow bedsit, before I met my first husband, Raymond.

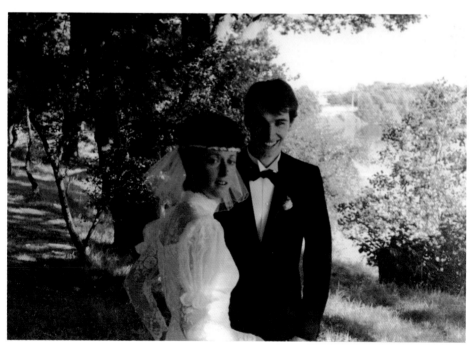

With Raymond on our wedding day in 1986.

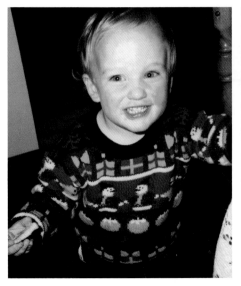
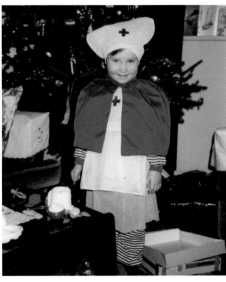

My blue-eyed boy, Michael, aged three, and four-year-old Siobhán looking pleased with her new outfit!

Me and my babies in 1996, shortly after my marriage breakdown.

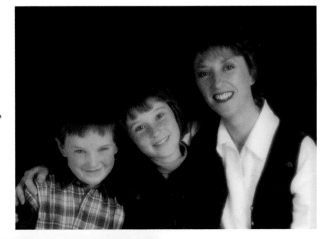

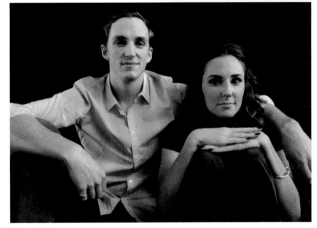

Michael and Siobhán, all grown up.

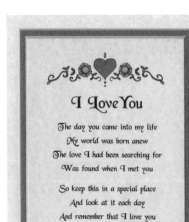

The beautiful poem that Daniel sent me on our wedding day.

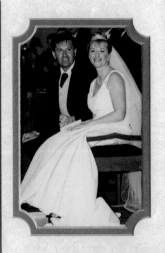

The two of us with Daniel's mother, Julia. *(Barry McCall)*

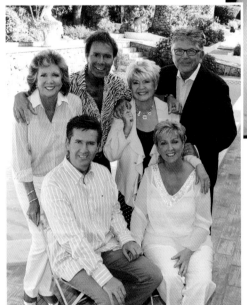

At Cliff Richard's house in Portugal, with Cilla Black, Gloria Hunniford and her husband, Stephen Way.

(Courtesy of VIP/Beta Bargartova)

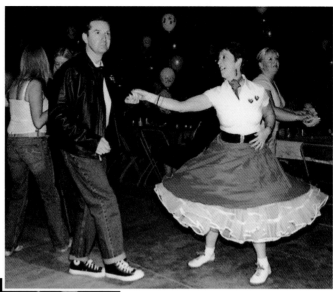

Fancy dress at the Donegal
Shore Festival in Kincasslagh:
nimble on our feet as we
dance rock 'n' roll, and well
disguised as hippies!

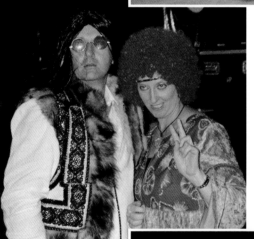

Singing on stage
with Daniel.

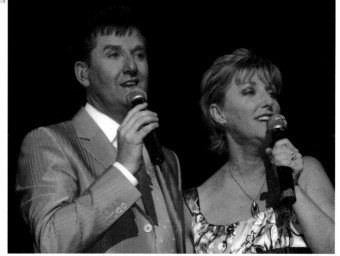

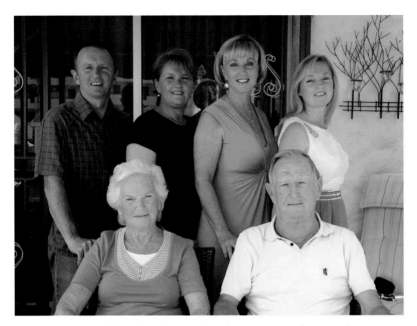

Family photo: with my brother Michael, sisters Josephine and Moira, and Mum and Dad.

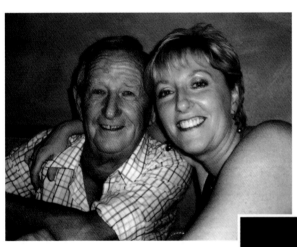

With my wonderful father Tom Roche, shortly before he died, and my equally wonderful husband Daniel – we just love dancing.

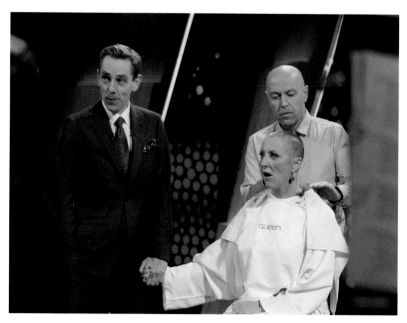

September 2013 and the moment I had my head shaved on live TV.
(Courtesy of the Irish Cancer Society)

Me with my
chemo bag.

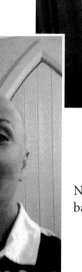

Not bad for a
bald woman!

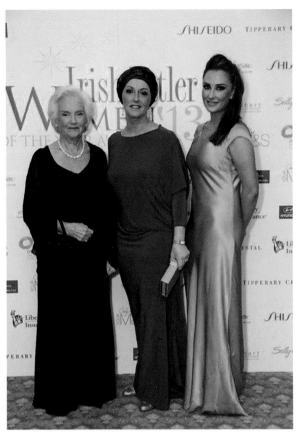

My beautiful mother Marion and daughter Siobhán at the Irish Tatler Awards ceremony, in November 2013.

(Courtesy of Irish Tatler Magazine)

The four of us: Siobhán and Michael with Daniel and me, at a family wedding in April 2014.

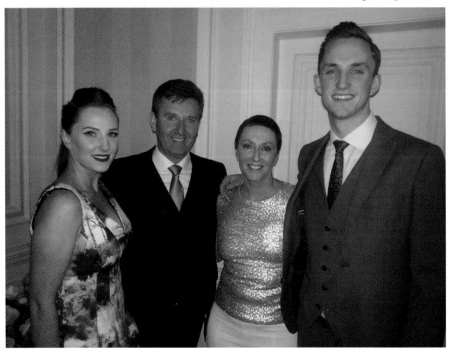

Raymond was working so hard and all I had to do was look after the children and I couldn't even do that. Anyway, that break did help and I never needed social services again. Strange that even they never mentioned the possibility of post-natal depression! Maybe it wasn't recognized so much back then.

Things were going from bad to worse with Raymond and me. I'm sure it wasn't easy coming home to someone as depressed as I was then. It's so hard for anyone who has not experienced it to understand just how awful depression can be. People don't know how to deal with it. They can't connect with you, so it frustrates them. The thing is, when you're depressed, it's almost impossible to connect with anyone! It's as if you're not really part of what's going on around you. Your body is there, but your mind is totally isolated from everything. You are totally alone, even though you may be in a room with hundreds of people. It's the loneliest place you can ever imagine, magnified one hundred times.

I had experienced depression before this, but this was different: much worse and more intense. Also, when I was younger and had depression, I could distract myself by changing where I lived, which I did a lot. I could decide to give up my job and get another one, or move from one town to the next. I suppose I was always trying to escape something, but this time I couldn't. I had a family, a husband and children who relied on me. I couldn't just get up and go. This time it had to be faced and dealt with – I had never experienced that before.

I was very low, but I also knew that my marriage problems were growing worse. Eventually, I asked Raymond if he would come to marriage counselling with me and he agreed. That was a great start because it meant that he wanted the marriage to work as much as I did. We got on fine, but it was useless, really, because Raymond was not being truthful about anything. He was saying what he thought he should say, but not what he actually felt. At one point, I asked Raymond to put his hand on his heart, to look me in the eye and to swear on his children's lives that he wasn't having an affair. He did exactly that! He looked me straight in the eye and said, 'I swear on our children's lives I am not having an affair'. Well, that was it. I was sure I was going out of my mind. As far as I was concerned, nobody would ever do something like that if it wasn't true, would they?

I was sure now that I was unstable, so I decided to see a psychologist to work on myself and to see what was causing me to think that my husband was having an affair. I had a few sessions with the psychologist and he asked if Raymond would come with me on one of my visits. He did and once again explained to the psychologist that he was very happy and that he couldn't understand why I thought he was having an affair. Nothing seemed to change between us. I knew we had made no progress whatsoever and I felt that there was nothing else that we could do to work things out, so we decided to have a break from the marriage. It wasn't as if we were arguing all the time, but it was as if we didn't connect any more. And what is the point of being with someone with whom you have no connection? I couldn't get him to talk to me about anything.

I was so unhappy and felt very alone. He was supposed to be my best friend, but he couldn't even talk to me and I felt that somehow, I was the cause of that. He told me years later that I pressed all the wrong buttons in him. It just disappointed me that he was never willing to try and work out those issues together and that it was easier for him to walk away.

Of course, at this stage I didn't realize that there were more than two of us in this marriage! I found this out when talking to my ex-boss, who Raymond had also worked for.

I told him that we were taking a break, but that there was no one else involved. To my surprise, he asked me if I was sure of that and I said I was absolutely sure. He then admitted that he had organized a hotel room for Raymond and one other for a weekend a few months previously. I couldn't believe it. I checked my diary to see what I had in it for that weekend and, sure enough, Raymond had been away on a business trip from that Friday to Sunday. I cannot even begin to put into words how physically sick I felt, knowing that he had been with someone else. My world fell apart.

I managed to get a copy of the hotel records, as I had previously worked there, and I went home that night, determined to get Raymond to tell me the truth. I knew that he would deny it, as he always had, which was why I had to have written proof.

He was in bed when I got home and I went into the bedroom and asked, once again, if he was having an affair. Of course, he denied it. I told him that I knew he was and that I had proof of it, but he just kept denying it, so I kept asking until, after about five hours, when I had worn him out, he admitted it. My initial thought was one of utter relief. 'Thanks be to God I am not going out of my mind,' was all I could say, followed by a string of abuse. I felt physically sick to my stomach and experienced a huge feeling of betrayal. I knew then that even if we managed to sort things out, my life as I knew it had changed for ever. That wonderful fairytale story I thought I was living was gone and would never be the same again.

I knew the girl he was having the affair with, so I immediately went to her house – it was now seven o'clock in the morning. She reluctantly let me in and I asked her if she loved my husband. She replied that she did, so I told her that she was welcome to him and his dirty socks and underwear and that I would drop the kids to her on Friday evenings and collect them after school on Monday. That way they could spend their weekends with their father. I mean, fair is fair. I sounded confident, even aggressive, but of course I didn't feel that confident at all. It was all a front on my part. I was falling to pieces and I could not believe that my husband was in love with someone else.

Raymond was all I ever thought about and while I was married to him, I would never have even dreamed of kissing another person, never mind sleeping with them! I was sure that he felt the same and that he had the same principles as me with regard to fidelity. We were four years married at this stage and, up to the point where I began to suspect that he might be having an affair, I honestly believed that I was the luckiest girl in the world. I had a husband and two lovely children, and my life had seemed perfect.

Raymond moved out of the house, although I don't think his relationship with her lasted very long after that. Maybe the idea of being a weekend mum to two children didn't sit with her very well. I asked Raymond several times why he had the affair, but I never got a satisfactory answer. Maybe having two young children and a wife was more difficult than he thought it would be. Personally, I think he liked the thrill of a new relationship and to know that he was still able to 'pull' the women, but I was devastated, to say the least. How could I go on and survive on my own with two young children, I wondered. I had never wanted to be a single parent because I knew that it would be very tough and I didn't think I had the strength to cope with it. I didn't know if I would make a good parent on my own. Now, I had no choice. I *was* on my own and there was nothing I could do to change that. I hated it. I cried and cried until the eyes in my head were swollen.

Even though Raymond had had the affair, I wanted him back, even though I was always the one who said that I would never put up with a man cheating on me! You really never know how you will react in any situation until you are in it. I wanted to be a family again. I missed the company and I thought that if I was a better wife, he would want me back again.

Raymond and I met at a party about three months later, in February 1991, and ended up together again. He never really said sorry for the affair, but I was just so glad to have him back that I didn't care. I was desperate for that security. We decided that we would move to Ireland and make a fresh start and put the past behind us. Raymond had the opportunity to work in Dublin later that year and I thought this was a great idea because everybody we knew in Edinburgh knew about the affair at this stage and in Ireland, we could have a clean slate.

However, things didn't really change and it wasn't long before Raymond had another affair and I moved out of our rented house with the kids. Even so, I *still* hoped that he would miss us and want us back. We played at being together, but he was not really interested in making a go of it. Before long, there was another woman. This one was French and he was really into her. Their behaviour at the time really hurt. I was, after all, the mother of his children and yet he didn't seem to care how hurt I was, as long as she was happy. Yet, even while he was going out with this woman, we ended up in bed together and I still believed he might come back. This was all happening in the first couple of years after the initial affair in Edinburgh. I realized that he was like a drug to me. I would go for a few weeks without wanting to be with him and I would be feeling strong and then we would end up in bed and I knew that I would have taken several steps back in my recovery. What is it they say, 'two steps forward, one step back'. That was me. Then I would be really angry with myself because I would realize that he had no intention of coming back to me. I felt that I was just someone that was there for the taking, so to speak. You see, I couldn't imagine myself with anyone else and it felt very natural to be with Raymond, bad though it was, so it was easy to slip back. I did that a few times, but the gaps got longer and longer each time, before I decided that this was it. No more.

I now know that nothing I could have done would have made Raymond stay in the marriage. We were just not meant to be together. I can see that very clearly now that I am married to Daniel and I know what a healthy relationship is like. It seemed to be a constant struggle being married to Raymond, but that is not the case with Daniel. We seem to just flow along through life together. Daniel is a wonderful gift that God has given me and I am so thankful for him every day.

So, Raymond and I decided to get divorced and go our separate ways. Once again, I decided to move. This time, it was back to Edinburgh because I couldn't bear the thought of seeing Raymond with this other woman. I wanted to be well away from them. God forgive me, but I remember thinking at that time that it would have been so much easier if he had died. People would be offering their support instead of telling me to 'get on with it'. 'You're lucky to be rid of him'; 'He was only a womaniser anyway', were the kinds of things people would say. If Raymond died, I thought, I would get insurance, so my finances would be better and, most importantly of all, I would never have to see him with another woman again. If he died, his leaving would not reflect on me personally, but leaving me for another woman was a total rejection of me as a person and that hurt beyond belief. Let me make it clear that I didn't wish Raymond any harm. I wasn't thinking clearly at all at this stage.

I was never good at being alone and now I had endless nights after the children were in bed feeling so lonely and rejected. I was working full time at this stage and I found it hard trying to do my job well *and* being a good mum. I had my wages coming in, but I found it tough trying to watch the pennies all the same. I would go into the supermarket with a few pounds and I would always take a calculator with me, so that I would never spend more than I had. I was proud like that and I would have hated to hand back something because I was short of money. The weekends were particularly lonely because I wouldn't have the interaction with my work colleagues. I would have to prepare for the following week by washing uniforms and clothes and doing the food shop and the usual things that needed doing. I never had enough money to go out, so every now and then a couple of girlfriends would come around and we would have a bottle of wine or two. I felt like an empty shell, just existing from day to day.

I began to read a lot of 'self-help' books then, which were a bit of an eye-opener. I knew that I had to learn to be alone and to be happy that way. I knew that my need to have a man in my life was unhealthy because I believed I couldn't be happy without one. I read more and more on the subject and I went on a few courses run by a man called Jack Black, who is the founder of an organisation called 'MindStore'. It runs personal development and performance programmes and I found them very beneficial. I seemed to 'get' what he was talking about and this was all helping to make me a stronger person in the long run. And it *was* in the long run. I am not talking about changing overnight. I didn't just read a book or go on a course and think I was all sorted. It was a long, slow process, but I was getting there.

Even though all of this turmoil was going on for so long, I tried very hard to keep Siobhán and Michael as sheltered from it as I possibly could. Raymond and I decided that when we were divorcing, we would talk to them and be as honest as we could about what had happened, taking their ages into consideration. I know that all the moving was probably not a good start for them, but it was the best that I could do at the time. Children are very adaptable and I knew that they would be OK. I made sure that I never fought with Raymond in front of the children, so they never really saw any conflict between us. If you ask Siobhán and Michael now how they felt during that period, they would say that they never really noticed anything and all the moving was very normal to them. They say that they can't even imagine Raymond and I as a couple, which is funny really. Even at the early stages of our marriage troubles, when Siobhán was about seven, I asked her if she would like Mum and Dad to be together again and she said no. I asked her why and she said: 'Because Daddy would only hurt you again.'

*

When Siobhán and Michael were young, we talked about them going to boarding school as Raymond had attended Fettes College in Edinburgh and he wanted the kids to go there, too. When the time came, we talked to Siobhán, who was at this stage twelve years old, and she really wanted to go. I had no objections as I had spent a year in boarding school and I had really enjoyed it. As the plans were being made for her to go, Michael protested that it was unfair that he wasn't going, too. I explained that he was very young at ten years old, but he kept on and on and eventually we gave in and he joined Siobhan in boarding school. I have to say that they loved it. They enjoyed the social aspect to it and all the friends they made and the facilities it provided. I was happy with them being there because after all the moving that they had done up to that stage, I felt they were getting the stability in life that they needed. Now they were happy and they could stay there until they left school, if that's what they wanted.

However, this left me feeling rather redundant as a parent and on the long evenings on my own, I felt that my life was going nowhere. I tried to go out and meet people, but I really wasn't interested in the pub scene and the drunken guys who would only approach you at the end of the evening, when they were incoherent. I hadn't been out with anyone since my marriage breakdown, which was about four years previously, and I was fed up with just existing. After everything that had happened over the previous few years, I decided that I wanted more from life. I wanted to feel alive, happy, worthwhile and safe. I needed to take time for myself and to get away from all the pressures I was feeling. At this time, my parents were living in Tenerife, having bought a bar there, and so I gave up my job, decided I would rent my house out in Edinburgh and move to Tenerife for a couple of years. It was time for a change.

Chapter 6

WHAT I LEARNED AND HOW I CHANGED

I am a very different person nowadays to the person I was before I married Raymond, and that's a good thing because I was very needy and I had given control of my self-worth and happiness to other people. I was constantly looking for love and to be loved. I didn't know how to be on my own and to be happy. I don't think I would ever have found happiness had I not looked at myself and changed some fundamental things about me as a person. I learned that you can never truly be loved by someone else until you have learned to love and respect yourself. I started that journey when my life was catapulted in a direction that I wasn't expecting.

I was devastated when my marriage broke down and at

that time I would have been happy if my life had ended. I genuinely felt that my family would be better off without me, including the children. I thought that their father could bring them up and that they wouldn't have to put up with this neurotic person, who was constantly miserable. I felt that it was my fault that their father had left and the guilt was almost too much to bear.

I hung on to the possibility that we would get back together for a long time after we had split. I was completely caught up in the past and unable to move on. I just couldn't see a future that I wanted to be in without my husband. Until I stopped looking back and learned to let go of the past, my life was at a standstill.

I hated Raymond for causing me so much pain. I hated him for leaving our children. I hated him for lying and cheating and disrespecting me, but I still couldn't let what I believed was my future go. I always seemed to be willing to give it another shot.

It took me some time to realize that I was disrespecting myself by constantly moving the boundaries of what was acceptable to me in our marriage. I had always said to myself that if my husband slept with someone else, I would forgive him once if it was a mistake. I rationalized it by telling myself that we all make mistakes and we should be given a second chance in life. So when Raymond had the initial affair, I forgave him. He had made a mistake, but then, when he made another one and another one, I just kept moving my boundaries of acceptability until I had none left and that is a bad thing to do. I was inviting him not to respect me because of my lack of respect for myself. That is a huge lesson that I have learned since then: you should always know what is acceptable to you in a relationship and stick to it.

During the time when we were separating, Raymond visited the children regularly. I was very insistent on that because he was their father and I could never deny that. That was painful at times because they would come back and tell me things about him that I didn't want to hear. However, I made a very clear decision not to run Raymond down in front of the children. I wanted the break-up to be as painless for them as possible. He may have been a bad husband to me, but he was a good father to the children. The relationship between a husband and wife is just that. It is between the two of them only and just because you are pissed off with your partner doesn't mean that you have to involve your children.

We still had to reach a financial settlement at the time, but that didn't matter to me because I was very proud and

I figured that if I wasn't good enough for him and he didn't want me, then I wanted nothing from him either. I see and hear of plenty of women who want to fleece their husbands when they have had affairs to make them pay for their mistakes, but I never felt like that. The fact that he rejected me made me feel so useless and worthless that I felt that taking anything else from him at that stage would be to lower myself even further. I figured that in time, he would realize that it was his loss to have missed so much of their formative years and surely that would be punishment enough. That rationalisation may seem strange, but that's how I felt. I didn't hide the fact that their father was with someone else, but I was never nasty about it to them. I always thought that when the children would grow up, they would make up their own minds about the type of people Raymond and I both are. My trying to destroy him in their eyes could very easily backfire in the long run.

Now that they are older, they both know what each of our strengths and weaknesses are. They come to me for some things and they go to Raymond for others. Another thing I learned was that you have to be a very bad parent for your children not to love you. I remember thinking that I was so great because I had been faithful and I was the one who had brought the children up, so I should get brownie points for that in their eyes, but it doesn't work like that. My children love Raymond and me equally and, at first, that was hard to accept. I expected them to understand how much he had hurt me and I suppose to be a bit angry with him for that but, as I said earlier, that was my problem, not theirs, and I am very proud that they never let that affect their relationship with their dad.

All in all, I am happy with the way in which I conducted myself when my marriage broke down. Apart from a few moments of madness, I continued to be reasonable and objective most of the time and I'm glad to say that it has certainly been worth it. My children have very little memory of those bad times; in fact, they can't even remember a time when we were together as a family and, as I said before, they find the thought of Raymond and I as a couple very strange indeed. He has since remarried a nice Scottish-Italian woman called Teresa and they have two beautiful children. Siobhán and Michael think the world of them and although it does feel strange that my son and daughter have a sister and brother that have nothing to do with me, I am delighted that they are so close.

*

Of course, at the time my marriage broke down, all of this was in the future. In the aftermath of the breakdown, I was extremely unhappy and I suffered a lot with depression. I knew that I needed to do something about it. I needed to try and understand why I was so unfulfilled and why my marriage had failed. What part did I play in its demise? How could I guard myself against that kind of hurt again? How could I learn to trust again? I had so many questions that I needed answers to. Raymond had had the affairs, but I felt that he was not really interested in saving the marriage and I couldn't understand that. We had two beautiful, very young children and I just didn't know how he could walk away from them. I thought that I must have been a really bad person for him to be able to leave and I felt a huge lack of self-worth.

I decided to meet with a psychologist once a week to talk about what I was feeling and thinking. This was a different psychologist to the one I had seen before, and she was wonderful. She guided me to a new way of seeing things. I remember one time she recommended a book to me and she asked me to read it before our next meeting. It was called *Codependent No More* by Melody Beattie, a brilliant book about how we define ourselves in terms of our relationships with others and try to 'control' them. When I met the psychologist for our next session, she asked me if I had seen myself anywhere in the book and I said, 'No. I am *everywhere* in the book'. She said that she was so glad because if I hadn't recognized my behaviour, I wouldn't have been ready to change; you first need to realize and accept how you are behaving to be able to change it. I was what is known as a 'Fixer', the type of person that wanted to 'fix' people, and there are lots of us about! You find someone with problems and you feel sorry for them, then you convince yourself that you can help them with their problems, for example, an alcoholic. You believe that if you are understanding enough and you help them and support them, that they will see the light and change. Wrong!! It's impossible to change anyone but yourself. A person has to want to change themselves. Yes, you can support them, but only in healthy ways and always with boundaries.

Another book I read at this time was called *The Dance Of Intimacy* by Harriet Lerner. I found it very interesting because it talked about the concept of two people in a relationship almost being like a dance: if you change direction, then the other person must change, too. You cannot change them, but if you change how you behave, or dance, their reaction to you will automatically change in response. It is so true and I have experienced that with my own father. As a child, I feared him and by the time I was thirty-six years old, I still felt the same. I spent all my life trying to impress him and to make him acknowledge his love for me and when he didn't treat me in the way I would have liked, I never said a word or pulled him up on it. I 'allowed' him to behave towards me the way he did. So the 'dance' continued for many years without change. Once I started doing courses and reading books on the subject, I started to change my behaviour towards him. The result was amazing: my father's behaviour towards me started to change in response. I learned to stand up to him and to tell him in no uncertain terms when I felt he was disrespecting me. I realized that, just because he was my father didn't mean that he was always right. I was an adult now and my feelings mattered.

It was hard at the beginning because I was afraid to stand up to him, although I really don't know what I was afraid of. He had never in his life been physically abusive towards me, but I was still scared. Slowly but surely, I did stand up to him and he respected me more for it. We ended up having a great relationship for the last fifteen years of his life. Anyway, it's an interesting concept. If you changed your 'Dance of Intimacy' with your loved one, how would they react in response?

*

When I attended the MindStore courses, what I learned helped me to focus on what I wanted in life and to think more positively about my life in general. I set goals that I wanted to achieve and for the first time in a very long time, I could see a future for myself. I learned that you have to plan for your future, regardless of what your position in life is. You need a map, so to speak, so that you can live your life with a purpose. If you don't have a purpose in life, you have nothing to aim for, nothing to keep you going, nothing to give you a sense of achievement, which is so important for your self-esteem. To constantly strive towards your purpose, you need to set yourself little goals. However, goal-setting is challenging and needs to be reviewed regularly to keep you on track.

I discovered that my purpose in life is to be contented, happy and healthy and to die knowing that my presence on this earth made a difference to another human being. To help me achieve my purpose, I set myself some goals. Nowadays, I have big goals and as life throws things at me, I have little or more immediate goals. For example, one of my big goals has been to set up a charity in Donegal to help people with depression and work on that has already begun. It is a long-term goal and will take some time to fully realize. A smaller or more immediate goal is to do an hour's walk four days a week to help to prevent cancer from rearing its ugly head again. They are just two examples of what I would consider a big and a little goal. The first goal will, I hope, make a difference to another human being and my second goal will help to keep me healthy.

Up to the point of my marriage breakdown, I always thought that it was someone else's job to make me happy, but since I have adopted this way of life, I have been far more content in myself. Before, if I wasn't happy, then it was because of what someone else had done. My wellbeing, both physically and mentally, was outside of my control. I now know that this doesn't have to be the case, but I also know how common it is: how many of us blame others for our misfortunes? I learned that I had to take responsibility for my own actions and their consequences. Blame is futile and achieves nothing. Now, when something goes wrong or something hurtful happens to me, of course, my first reaction is to give out and complain, but once I have calmed down, the first thing I want to do is sort out the problem if I can and if I can't, then I try to let it go. I'm not saying that it's easy, but it's what I try to do. Endless blaming and complaining is very negative and it takes so much energy that is needed for more important things, like fighting illness.

At the risk of sounding a bit wacky, I now believe that

we can do so much more in our lives if we try to be as positive as we can, to take responsibility for our own actions and to just get back in touch with the natural world we live in. Nowadays we are completely taken up with computers, iPads, mobile phones and technology in general. I actually had a row with Siobhán two Christmases ago because she was on the phone all of Christmas day and I felt it was an intrusion into our family time and space. She wasn't living in the present and enjoying what was going on around her. She was too busy texting friends and checking Facebook to see if she had missed anything. As far as I could see, what she was actually missing was Christmas day with her family, talking, playing games, watching a movie or whatever, but at least doing it together. Of course, she didn't see it like that and just thought that I was being a pain, but that's what we have to put up with as mothers! Some day she will understand what I was talking about. Maybe when she has her own children.

I believe that we need to be present in the moment. What I mean by that is that we should be aware of what we are doing at the minute and not constantly looking at what has been or will be. We only have this minute in our lives. We can't live in the past because its already gone and we can't live in the future because it hasn't arrived, so we can only live in the now. I know that everybody has heard that before, but how many of us actually practise it? How many of us actually cherish each moment we have? It's a difficult thing to do and it takes a lot of practice and sometimes I forget and I slip back into the old ways, but as soon as I am aware of what I am doing, I bring myself back to the present moment.

I learned through all of these experiences that we are all going through life doing the best that we can at any given moment. I think we all change a little with every experience we have and we grow as people because of it. I believe that everything happens for a reason and, as I look back on my life, I am glad for everything that I have gone through because I think I am a better person as a result. I used to be very set in my beliefs, but now I tend to be more open. The older I get, the more I realize I have so much still to learn and that humbles me. For example, I love a really good debate on lots of subjects but, unfortunately, I can come across as very ... passionate! Others might call it intense, feverish, fiery or even aggressive. I believe that if someone disagrees with me, or has another point of view, they should convince me to rethink my belief. If they manage that, then I will indeed be happy to reconsider. (That doesn't happen very often though ...) I think it is important to put yourself into another person's shoes before you judge them outright. Again, that isn't always easy to do, but I think, if we want to be compassionate towards others, we have to try and understand where they are coming from.

A good example of this comes with something that I saw at one of the MindStore courses that I attended. Two friends met after a party, where they had both been introduced to a girl they hadn't met before. One said to the other: 'I really didn't like that girl we met on Saturday night. I thought she was very forward, sure of herself, opinionated and rude'.

'Really?' said the other girl. 'That's weird, because I thought she was friendly, confident, assertive and a little cheeky.'

Neither person was wrong. They just saw her traits in different ways. Someone who is able to approach a stranger and talk to them may be seen as 'forward' or as 'friendly', depending on who's judging them. Someone who is 'sure of herself' may also be seen as 'full of it' and so on. There is no right or wrong. We just are as we are and that is why I believe in being myself. We all want to be liked but, regardless of how we behave, in general roughly fifty percent of people will like us and fifty percent won't. You can never please everyone all the time, so why not please yourself?

And I don't mean pleasing yourself at the expense of others! I used to try to be accepted by people and do whatever I thought would please them, but now I know that as long as I am true to myself, then some people will accept me and others won't. I can live with that.

I will never again feel the way I did when my marriage broke down because I am a different person now. I am much stronger and I can happily live on my own. I don't fear being alone any more. That was one thing that I always thought I could never do. I don't fear being rejected any more either. I can compromise, but I will never change to suit someone else just because I'm afraid to be left on my own. If I did end up on my own for whatever reason, I would survive. I know this because I survived through the worst of times. I know that I would get on with my life. It's not what I would choose, but I could handle it. It's amazing the power and strength that I get from knowing that. From knowing that everything will be OK.

I had absolutely no idea how to take control of my life when I was younger and that caused me a lot of unnecessary misery. Now, I have the know-how to take control of things. I know that I have a choice, even if the choices are difficult. I know that I can choose to walk if I am unhappy and that nobody else will ever have that control over me again. I remember something that the psychologist said to me once when I was complaining about my marriage to Raymond and I will never forget it. 'Majella, you are like a butterfly on the backside of an elephant. All you have to do is fly away.' I think what she meant was, 'Stop complaining about your situation and start doing something about it.' Up to this day, I hate to hear people complain about something, while they continue to accept it. If you're unhappy, then change something. Another great saying is, 'If you keep on doing what you've always done, then you'll keep on getting what you've always got.' How true that is.

I had some very difficult experiences in my life, but I wouldn't change them for the world. I am who I am because of what I have been through and because of what I have learned. I am very happy with the person I have become. I have grown so much and I don't feel as helpless as I did when I was younger. I love being in my fifties and I wouldn't want to be in my twenties for anything. You definitely have a greater confidence as you get older. I don't think it's that you know what you want from life, but you certainly know what you don't want. You aren't as affected by your peers as you were when you were young. You're not willing to put up with crap in your life any more. Well, I'm not anyway!

But back to my life then. It was about to change dramatically with my move to Tenerife in 1999 and I was well equipped, with all the mistakes I had made and the lessons I had learned from those mistakes, to hopefully make a better go of things than I had in the past. Little did I know that I was about to meet the absolute love of my life and, thankfully, I was emotionally healthy enough to realize it.

Chapter 7

DANIEL

There is something wonderful about waking up in the morning to a beautiful blue sky and I loved that about my first few months in Tenerife. It lifted my spirits no end. Of course, it was lovely to be around Mum and Dad, too, as, for the first time in ages, I felt looked after by people who cared about me. My parents had moved to Tenerife in 1991 and had a bar/restaurant in the south of the island. I was able to put my catering experience to good use and to help them in the day-to-day running of the place. I was relieved that I didn't have the pressure of my previous job and the sunshine certainly helped with my depression.

I began slowly to find my feet. I got an apartment of my own and during the school holidays, the children would come out to spend the time with me. I loved the life that Tenerife had to offer. The apartment that I moved into was outside the main tourist area, in the small village of Adeje. It is a typically Spanish village. In the morning I would walk to the local bakery to get fresh bread and maybe sit outside one of the numerous cafés for a cup of coffee. I love people-watching and what better way to do it than sitting in the sun, drinking coffee, watching the world go by.

I always tried to speak Spanish whenever I could and I managed to make myself understood most of the time, but when the locals spoke back to me, I was lost. I hadn't a clue what they were saying! I haven't improved much since then, even though I did spend three weeks in Spain, where I took an intensive Spanish course. It was so intensive that, by the time I finished the course, I didn't even know how to say 'hello' in Spanish! My brain had completely seized up. I took in as much as I could and then, all of a sudden, everything was gone. It was as if I had overdosed on the language. However, I think some of what I learned did sink in because every now and then I will come out with a Spanish word and I have no idea where it came from. Obviously, it is just there in my brain somewhere. But it was important for me to try to learn, so that I could fit in.

Mum and Dad had a lot of Irish friends in Tenerife, so they had a pretty good social life. There were a lot of people who had their own apartments and spent maybe two or three months a year there during the winter. I found that the work in the bar was easy because all it really involved was serving people and chatting with them. It was so different from what I had been used to and I was so glad to get away from all the pressures I'd had when I was in Edinburgh. I was beginning at last to find my feet but, little did I know, things were about to change again.

One particular evening, when I was working at the bar, my mother told me that Daniel O'Donnell was coming in that night. I knew who Daniel O'Donnell was, although I didn't know him well at all. He had met my mother and father a few years previously, when a couple of their friends had brought him to their bar. From then on, whenever Daniel was visiting Tenerife, he would always pop in to say hello to Mum and Dad. When my mother mentioned that he'd be visiting, I remembered that a few years previously, when I was on holidays, I had actually met him briefly. He had called in to ask after Mum and Dad and as they weren't there, we'd chatted for a bit, before he left.

I think most Irish people know who Daniel O'Donnell is because he has appeared on television many times and he's a bit of an Irish icon. I knew that he was a nice guy and I was certainly interested in meeting him again, but I wasn't into his music and I had never seen him perform, so I suppose I had some misconceptions about what he would be like. From what I had heard and seen of him myself, I thought that he would be very quiet and probably quite boring. I thought that the type of music he was into meant that we would have nothing in common. In my teens, I had listened to people such as Janis Ian, the Eagles, Queen, Carole King, James Taylor and many others, but I had never listened to any Irish artists.

That night, he arrived with a couple of friends and he had something to eat. I was introduced to him and sat at his table for a little while. The bar was particularly quiet that night and Mum was a little bit concerned that Daniel might not enjoy his evening. We didn't have any entertainment in the bar, so Mum said, 'Why don't you sing something?' One of my party pieces is the ballad, 'She Moved Through the Fair'. We didn't have a stage or anything like that, so I just stood in the middle of the bar and off I went. It was strange to be singing for a singer, but I wasn't doing it to be judged, so it didn't bother me. As I always say, it's only a bit of fun, not a performance. You can take yourself too seriously sometimes.

I didn't really sing much at that stage, only in a pub with a few drinks if a sing-song got underway. I remember when I moved to London first, I was at a party and I asked when the music would be turned off, so we could have a sing-song. Everyone looked at me as if I had two heads, but that was what I was used to. That's what we did at parties at home in Ireland. I decided I would sing anyway, as I'd had a few drinks and the courage was mighty, but everyone started to make smart comments and jokes, so I just stopped. That finished my singing in London for a long time.

I think I introduced the song by saying that he was always singing for other people, so tonight, I was going to sing for him and then, bold as brass, I belted out my version of the song. He thought it was lovely, but then again, what else could he say? Daniel was hardly going to say that I was rubbish! We chatted some more and I had my picture taken with him. We got on well and I found it very easy to talk to him. He was with another couple from home and as he was leaving, he asked if I would like to join them the following evening, as they were going to a place called Bobby's, which was in the centre of Playa de Las Americas. This surprised me, as Bobby's was a nightclub and really didn't start to get going until about one o'clock in the morning. I thought to myself that I had to see this: Daniel O'Donnell in Bobby's!

At this stage, I didn't have any thoughts about Daniel in a romantic way. I just didn't think it was on the cards. I thought he was a lovely guy and very funny, which surprised me, but as I was divorced with two children, I certainly didn't think he would be interested in me. In fact, being with him in that way never crossed my mind at all. However, I found that the next day I was thinking about meeting him and I was actually really looking forward to it. I don't know if Daniel felt the same or not after the first meeting. I think he liked my company all right, but I don't think he thought much further than that.

That night, the four of us went out and we had a great evening. We went to the Dubliner, which is a late-night Irish bar with really good live music and then we went on to Bobby's. We were dancing all evening and at one point, Daniel leaned across and kissed me. I was so surprised and taken aback, but I was also really pleased. I realized that I actually liked this man and that he wasn't at all what I'd thought. He was funny, chatty, lively and attentive. We danced all night and the fact that he doesn't drink was a real bonus, even though I'd thought it would be the opposite. I thought he would get bored in a club, but he doesn't. He doesn't need drink to enjoy himself, but he doesn't stop others from doing so. I thought that he might be no craic and the fact that I liked a drink might put him off, but none of that matters to Daniel. He really does live and let live. He has always allowed me to be the person I am and has never tried to change anything about me. It also helps that he has a great sense of humour.

For the next week, while Daniel was in Tenerife, we spent every day together. We just got on so well and I enjoyed his company very much. He was easy to be with and very kind and thoughtful and I found that so refreshing. When he was due to go back to Ireland, I felt sad because I was enjoying my time with him and I reckoned that was the end of it. I hoped it wasn't, but I thought there was too much 'stuff' in the way.

Over the next while, we called each other fairly regularly and wrote a couple of times. This was in September of 1999 and I was due to go back to Scotland to pick up the kids from boarding school for their Christmas holidays. As it happened, Daniel was performing in Brentwood in Essex around that time and I decided that it would be a good opportunity for me to see him in action, so to speak. I called him and told him that I would be coming through London on my way to Scotland and that I'd love to see him in concert. When I told him I'd be coming alone, I think I made him a bit nervous.

I met him at his hotel in the afternoon and then we went to the theatre for the show. I knew that people were looking at me, wondering who I was because Daniel wasn't the type of person to have strange women with him. He introduced me as a friend from Tenerife and left it at that. When I took my seat in the theatre, I was amazed at how many people were there. I think I spent most of the evening looking at the faces of people in the audience and watching their expressions as Daniel told stories, sang songs and did silly little moves with his hips throughout the evening. It was not at all what I would've expected. He had a beautiful voice, but not only that, he had a wonderful connection with the audience. It was something I had never seen before. He had the ability to make every person feel as though he was speaking to him or her directly. He had a lovely way of telling stories: even to this day, if Daniel tells a story I have heard many times before, he still manages to make me laugh. He truly has a unique gift. He is not just a good singer, but a brilliant entertainer as well.

When we went back to the hotel that evening, we were chatting about various things and generally catching up on our lives, when I had the strangest feeling. It came completely out of the blue and I couldn't explain it at all. I said to myself: 'I am going to marry this guy some day'. It wasn't a conscious decision; I wasn't taking control of my own destiny or anything like that. The point is, I felt that it *wasn't* in my control! It was going to happen and that was just a fact. It was as if I was being told by someone outside of me that this was going to happen in the future. I felt absolutely sure about it. I can assure you that this is not the sort of thing I would normally say to a man – I'm sure any man would run a mile if a woman told him that on their second proper date! Nonetheless, because I was absolutely one hundred per cent sure, I felt I had nothing to lose by telling him. And so I did. I told him straight out that I was going to marry him. I said, 'I know this makes me sound like a "bunny boiler", but I'm telling you, we are going to marry one day'. He was pretty taken aback, but he was polite, as always! I think he just said, 'Oh really'. He did tell me afterwards that he thought I was a bit mad. It certainly didn't encourage him to fall for me, that's for sure.

The following day I left to go to Scotland to pick up

Siobhán and Michael from boarding school and to bring them to Tenerife for Christmas. Daniel didn't return to the island again until about April of the following year, but we did speak regularly on the phone. I can still remember the day I was to pick him up from the airport when he came out in April 2000. I was so excited at the thought of seeing him again that I just felt like a fifteen-year-old. We had another wonderful week together but, as usual, it was all too short and, before I knew it, he was leaving again. But we seemed to get a lot closer that week and the connection was definitely getting stronger all the time. We talked about so many things and shared some very intimate thoughts and beliefs. I never discussed the marriage thing again because I had no need to. I'd had that feeling when we met and I'd told him about it and that was it. If it was to become a reality, then it would in its own time.

Daniel must have done a lot of thinking over the next while and realized that things were getting quite serious. That probably scared him a little because the next time he came to Tenerife, things had changed and he seemed a little more distant than usual. One evening, we had been out for dinner and we went back to his apartment afterwards. He told me that he thought the relationship couldn't go any further and that he was really sorry, but hoped we could continue to be friends. As I had suspected, Daniel was very uncomfortable with the fact that I was divorced with children and he couldn't see how being with me could work for him.

I couldn't wait to get out of the apartment: I felt so vulnerable. He asked me if I was devastated and I said: 'No, Daniel. I'm not devastated. I was devastated when my husband left me with two very young children. I'm not devastated, but I am very disappointed'.

I didn't try to change his mind in any way. If someone wants to go, then you have to accept that. I had begged too many times in past relationships and that would never happen again. I knew that if he changed his mind, he would do so in his own time. Nonetheless, I left that evening and went home with my heart feeling very low. I suppose I had begun to think that being a couple could be a reality, but when he finished with me, I knew it was just a dream. However, I didn't fall apart as I had in previous relationships. That side of me was well and truly in the past. I was a much healthier person in that respect. I hated that it was over, but my life didn't depend on it as it had done in previous years.

Daniel called again a few days later and asked if I

wanted to come to a photo shoot that was taking place in Tenerife. I was a bit surprised because he'd finished with me, but I had said that I would be happy to be friends, so I went along. To be honest, it was very difficult for me, because I had well and truly fallen for him at this stage and every time I saw him, I wanted to be close to him. We did go out a few times during that visit, but always as friends and even though it wasn't easy, I knew that it would be OK in the end. I didn't know how, but I just knew it would be. I am not like that about everything. Sometimes I haven't a clue what to think or feel, but a bit like I knew the head shave was going to be OK, I knew that about Daniel and myself, too.

Even though we kept in touch over the months that followed, I missed the closeness that we had had as a couple. We still talked on the phone fairly regularly, but it wasn't the same. It's always nice when you have somebody in your life that you care about. It's exciting and you look forward to hearing from them and seeing them and sharing things with them. I was back to being alone again, but I got on with my life and my friends in Tenerife. I didn't really socialize very much and I probably only went out once or twice a week. I suppose I'm a bit of home-bird and I enjoy pottering about my house. It's nice to get dressed up every now and then and go out to have a good time, but only every now and then. I certainly wouldn't want to be doing it all the time. I find having to get myself all dolled up for an evening out is a real nuisance and, most of the time, I just can't be bothered. So, life was pretty quiet, as it is for most people and I just went to work every day and did the usual things that most people do. I had managed to build a life for myself on the island, with or without Daniel, and I knew that I'd be OK. I had done so much work on myself to this point that I knew I would never be as broken again over the loss of somebody. I was happy in Tenerife and I enjoyed the life there. It was all a bit of an adventure as I knew I wouldn't be there for ever – I could relax and enjoy myself for a bit.

The following September, Daniel was back in Tenerife again. As usual, I picked him up from the airport and we went back to his apartment. He told me that he had been thinking about me and that he couldn't understand why, in the strangest of places, I would pop into his head. He said he'd given it a lot of thought and that he enjoyed my company and loved being with me and that he didn't think God would want to deny him the love he had found. Of course, I was delighted to hear this as I totally believed that, too. I knew that Daniel had had difficulties with his religion and our relationship. He is a practising Catholic and wants to do the best he can in the eyes of God. I do, too, but I don't believe that the rules made by the Catholic institution are necessarily always right. And if I don't agree with them, then I look for guidance in other ways. Surely love always comes from a good place? I wanted Daniel to trust that things would work out between us and that we would make a great team. I felt that he would have a happier life and I wanted him to believe that and trust in it and not dismiss it because the church said it was wrong. We decided we would give it our best shot and deal with whatever difficulties that came our way as they occurred.

I wondered how Daniel's mother would feel about him getting together with a divorced woman who had two children. I suppose if he had been my son, I would have been concerned. She didn't know who I was or what my intentions were and I suppose she might have thought that I would take advantage of Daniel. After all, he was a very eligible, wealthy single man and I'm sure she was hoping that one day he would meet a nice single Irish girl, settle down and have a family. I was forty-one at this stage, so the chances of us having a family were fairly limited.

Julia came to Tenerife on one occasion and we got on

very well. I think what she said to Daniel was, 'She's a worker', and coming from her, that was very high praise. Julia wouldn't have had much time for women who spend all their time painting their nails, putting on make-up and having their hair done. That was not the era or life that Julia came from. She saw that I was a hands-on kind of person. If something needs doing, then I'll give it my best shot, even if I end up messing things up. I figure that you won't learn anything if you don't at least try. So, when she was staying with us she saw that I was wiring plugs, tuning in televisions, painting and doing whatever needed doing. I think she admired that in me.

However, Julia was very close to Daniel and I certainly didn't want to come between them. Daniel had great respect for his mother and always spoke very highly of her and I respected that. He has been referred to as a 'Mammy's boy', but I see that as a very positive thing. Most men think that their mothers are wonderful: the difference is that Daniel isn't afraid to say it. That makes him a bigger man in my eyes.

When Julia was a young woman, the qualities a man would look for in his future wife would've been very different to what they are today. She would have needed to be a good housekeeper, to be able to roll her sleeves up and get stuck into whatever work needed doing. She would need to be good to her husband, to feed him well and to look after the children. That was her duty and that was what was expected of her. I can totally understand that, but things are very different these days. People expect other things from marriage now, compared to seventy years ago. Nowadays, we want our partners to understand us emotionally. We want them to care about what makes us happy in life. We want them to encourage us to fulfil our ambitions and when we are vulnerable, we want them to be there for us and to support us. Where Julia came from, people were too busy just trying to survive. They worked the land from morning till night. They had no running water or electricity, so everything they did was difficult. The men spent their days fishing when the weather would allow, going to the bog to get turf for their fires, looking after the animals and, in the winter, they mended their fishing nets or many of them went to Scotland to find work. Most houses only had two rooms and most families had at least four children. There would've been no privacy whatsoever. Their lives were very simple, but also very happy. I sometimes wonder whether they were better off in those days.

*

Julia passed away on 18 May 2014. She would have been ninety-five in the July. She was an amazing woman right up until her death. She had a very sharp mind and liked to be involved in all her children's lives. We got on well, even though we had our differences at times and I think that she knew that I love her son very much and that I try to be the best partner I can be and to support him in whatever way I can. That's all a mother wants to know, that her child is happy.

Thankfully, Daniel was at home for a few days before Julia passed away. He was glad that he had the time to spend with her. Two of her grandchildren and one of their girlfriends were with her when she passed away. It was about 4.20 in the morning and Daniel and I raced up to the hospital when we got the call. She was still warm and, for a moment, I wondered if she was really gone because she just looked like she was sleeping. Daniel was obviously very upset, but he was glad that she wasn't suffering any more and that she was now with Francie, her husband, after all the years they'd been apart. He had died in 1968 at only forty-nine years of age.

Julia was waked in her home for two nights, which is very normal in Donegal. When we saw her in the coffin, she looked as if she was sleeping. She had not failed in anyway. Maybe that's a Donegal saying, but what I mean is that she didn't look any different than in the previous few years. She hadn't had a long illness that would have taken so much out of her. She had lovely clothes on and her hair was fixed and her face was made up. She looked lovely, but I felt very sad when I saw her because I thought of my father, wrapped in a sheet, looking awful, and then he was gone. I wished that we'd had a wake for Dad. It's such a healthy thing. It gives you the chance to pray for the person and to talk about their lives and to reminisce about the good and bad times. We got the chance to spend time with Julia's remains and to give ourselves time to realize that she was gone. It just wasn't like that with Dad.

While Daniel and I were seeing each other, we tried to keep it as quiet as possible. We knew that if the media found out about us, it would be reported in the paper and it would put extra pressure on the relationship when we were really just trying to get to know each other. If that had happened, the relationship would've been over before it had really begun. We had been involved for about six months at this stage, but if we went out together people wanted photos. We tried to behave as friends rather than as a couple. As the months went on, I visited Daniel on a few occasions and we were always on the phone to each other. We both knew that we would make a good team and after about a year-and-a-half, we talked about the possibility of getting married. I was forty when I met Daniel and he was thirty-eight. We weren't teenagers and we really didn't see any point in dating each other for a long period.

Our relationship moved onto a different footing in early December 2001, when Daniel turned forty and a big party was held for him at the The Hilton Hotel, Birmingham, and tickets were sold for charity. It was a formal dinner and one thousand people attended, mainly fans of Daniel, other entertainers and close friends and family. At this stage, the public still didn't know about me and I was expecting to sit anonymously at a table with some of our friends. However, about an hour before dinner, Daniel announced that he was going to introduce me to the crowd as his girlfriend and that I would be sitting at the top table with the rest of his family. I went into a panic because I hadn't been expecting this at all and I hadn't had time to prepare myself. I knew that it would make the front page of the newspaper back home and I wasn't sure if I was ready to be launched into the public eye. I also remember that I was wearing a pretty low-cut dress that night and all I thought was, if he had told me he was going to introduce me, I would never have worn this dress! I felt so self-conscious because I knew all eyes would be on me. Everyone would be wondering who I was, where I came from, what he saw in me and what I had to offer. Would I change him? Would he become less available to all his fans? All those thoughts were going through my head and I felt sick.

I phoned my mother and I told her that everyone was going to know about us in a few hours. I told her that there would probably be stuff in the newspaper and that people might even want to talk to her and Dad about me. Daniel and I decided then that before the newspapers started making up their own stories, we would invite a reporter called Eddie Rowley, who was also a good friend and attending the dinner that night, to come and interview us in the hotel suite so that the article would appear in the paper the next day. At least then it would be an article that we were in control of and that we knew was going to be the truth.

When we walked into the room that night and I took my place next to Daniel at the top table, I felt as proud as punch. That was my first public appearance with Daniel and it was very nerve-wracking. Everybody was very kind, but I'm sure there must have been some people there who were wary of me and my intentions because they would have been very protective of Daniel. We had lots of pictures taken that evening, something that I was going to have to get used to if I was going to be a part of his life.

By this stage, we'd talked about marriage, but hadn't made any concrete plans. But by Christmas, all that was to change. I was having Christmas in Donegal in his house with his family and while I was getting the dinner ready, Daniel suggested that I go upstairs to the bedroom and call my mother and father in Tenerife to wish them a happy Christmas. I was a bit puzzled because I was in the middle of making dinner and his whole family was waiting, but when he insisted, I said OK. Little did I know!

I was sitting on the bed talking to my mother when Daniel came into the room and asked if he could speak to her. I gave him the telephone and after a bit of chat, he said, 'Do you know what I'm going to do now, Marion, I'm going to put a ring on your daughter's finger and I'm going to ask her to marry me.' I was flabbergasted and I started crying. I had no idea that he was going to do this or that he had bought a ring. Then my mother started crying! We went downstairs and told the rest of the family the news and I happily showed off my new engagement ring. Daniel had bought it for me while on tour in America the month before. It was a beautiful ring, and it would sit into the wedding band, which I really liked. At that point in time, I'm sure I was the happiest woman alive.

We decided to marry on Monday 4 November 2002. That was the only time that Daniel had off in between all his touring and even then, we had to go to America the day after the wedding so that he could start his annual round of concerts in Branson, Missouri. I really didn't mind. After all, I was forty-two years old, not twenty-two! All that mattered to me was that we would be married.

As I'd been a conference and banqueting manager, I was able to use my skills in organising the wedding myself. I'd had a fairly large wedding when I married Raymond and that hadn't worked out, so I wasn't really that concerned about that side of things. The most important thing to me was the ceremony and the fact that I was going to be Mrs Daniel O'Donnell. Of course, it was Daniel's first time and I wanted everything to be perfect for him. There were so many people that he wanted to invite and I was happy to fit in with whatever he wanted. We invited five hundred people and I think about fifty of those guests were people that I'd invited! As I said, all that was important to me was being married to Daniel. I wanted nothing to spoil that and, as far as I was concerned, the day couldn't come quick enough.

However, we still had one obstacle to overcome. At this point in time I was divorced and had applied to the Catholic Church for an annulment. It was very important to me to be able to marry in the church because although I am not very religious, I wanted to have God's blessing on such an occasion. I also knew how important it would be to Daniel to marry in the church and I felt guilty that I might deny him that opportunity.

I had spoken with a friend of mine who was a priest and he suggested that I apply for an annulment: because of the circumstances of the breakdown, he thought that I might be eligible. It was a fairly lengthy process with lots of members of our family being interviewed separately, including Raymond, and I have to say that I am very grateful that Raymond was honest about our marriage breakdown when he was being interviewed by the canon lawyers.

When the annulment was granted, Daniel and I were over the moon. Daniel had always wanted to marry in his local church, St Mary's in Kincasslagh, and that suited me perfectly because I had been living outside Ireland for the previous twenty years and most of my family lived in different parts of the world. I know that if I hadn't received the annulment, I would still be with Daniel and we would probably have married in a register office, however, I also know that he would never have been truly happy with that. He would've always felt that something was missing, so I was very happy to know that his wish was going to come true.

The run-up to the wedding went very smoothly and I was getting more and more excited as each day passed and we got closer and closer to 4 November. As I had been married before, I really wanted Daniel to have the wedding that he chose himself, but he wasn't bothered and said he would rather leave it to me, apart from the large guest list. That's just how it was. He had so many people to whom he meant something and who had helped him in the past and he really wanted them all to be there. I just wanted to be married, so I didn't mind. The church ceremony was the most important part for me. Of course I wanted a nice reception, but it really wasn't as important as it had been the first time around.

I bought my dress in America and I think it was the third dress I tried on, a traditional white satin with a simple sleeveless bodice, decorated with pearls. Again, it wasn't the dress that was important to me. That's the way I felt at the time, but if it was today, it would be a different matter. I would have been much choosier and more particular about the dress because it's now on display at the Daniel O'Donnell Visitor Centre in Dungloe. The centre houses all of Daniel's memorabilia, including gold and platinum discs and the various awards that he has received throughout the years. I did decide to have a long veil because I had never had one before, but it was all organized fairly quickly, so I really didn't have time to be pondering on ideas. Back then, I just wanted to be Mrs O'Donnell and nothing was as important as that.

When the day arrived, the weather was pretty bad, but I really didn't care. When I was getting ready, my mother told me that I was wanted at the front door. There was a man standing there with a small packet for me. He told me that it was from Daniel and I excitedly opened it up. It was a framed picture of the two of us with a beautiful poem entitled: 'The Day You Came Into My Life'. It was so romantic and I just melted and knew that I was about to marry a very special man. What a wonderful gesture. He also bought me a car, which just about blew me away – I think I bought him a St Christopher medal with the date inscribed on it! And I thought I was the romantic one ...

As was traditional, Daniel had been staying at his mother's house the night before the wedding. I called him to thank him for the gift and to tell him that I was the happiest woman alive to be marrying him that day. I had come so far in my journey and I really was a different person. Had I not been, then I would never have ended up with Daniel. I know that for sure. I know that I wouldn't have seen the wonderful person that he was either because I would have been too wrapped up in my own insecurities. This truly was a milestone in many respects.

When all the bridesmaids were ready, they all left the house, along with my mother. My father and I were the only two people left in the house. We got in the car to head for the church, but the electric gates to our house wouldn't open. We tried everything, but they just wouldn't budge. There were security men outside the gate and one of them had to go to the church to explain what the delay was. The funny thing was, it really didn't faze me in the least. As far as I was concerned, as long as I married Daniel, nothing could've gone wrong that day.

After about twenty minutes, we tried the remote control again and, this time, to our relief, the gate opened and off we went. I was so excited, but completely unprepared for the number of people waiting outside the church to see me. There were television cameras and reporters everywhere. I had had very little experience of the media up to that stage, so it was all very surreal for me.

When I got out of the car it was drizzling, but I wanted to go and shake hands with some of the people who had been waiting patiently in the rain. I was trying to hold my dress up so that it wouldn't get wet and at the same time trying to greet everyone. I was aware that I was very late at this stage, probably about half an hour, so I didn't hang about too long.

I will never forget how elated I felt as I stood at the top of the aisle with my father and the music started to play. We had the most wonderful autumnal flower displays all around the church, which I had organized with Alcorn's Flower and Garden Centre in Letterkenny. I had chosen Johann Pachelbel's 'Canon in D' as our processional music and as the first notes rang out, off we went. As I was walking down the aisle, I kept looking at Daniel to see if he would turn around but, to my surprise, he didn't. I was a bit disappointed as I'd hoped he would, but he explained to me afterwards that the priest had told him not to turn around and to wait to see me when I arrived by his side.

My dad walked me up the aisle and when we got to the top, he gave my hand to Daniel and said, 'Here she is, and I don't want her back this time!' He was always so witty and quick. We got a great laugh out of that later.

Daniel had chosen some of the music and some of the musicians in his band, John Staunton, Stephen Milne and Ronnie Kennedy, played, while Mary Duff, who sings with him, Trionagh Moore Allen and Leon McCrum did the singing. They were like angels. Daniel's sister Margaret, or Margo as she is known, is a well-known country singer and she sang a song called 'I Promise You', which has the most beautiful lyrics. It couldn't have been nicer. Father Brian D'Arcy conducted the ceremony along with our local parish priest, Father Pat Ward. Father Brian did a fantastic job of involving everyone throughout the ceremony.

When we left the church afterwards, all I could hear was the constant clicking of cameras and everyone asking us to look this way that way. It was all a bit of a frenzy. With the cameras flashing away, we got into the wedding car to head off to the reception in Letterkenny. It is only about forty-five kilometres away, but it took us about an hour and a half to get there. Normally it would only take about fifty minutes. Along the way, people were out in their gardens with banners, flags and messages of goodwill. I couldn't believe it. I felt like a superstar. Some people even had bonfires lit, as is tradition in the countryside. As we arrived into Letterkenny, there was a huge banner across the road, which said 'Congratulations to Daniel and Majella on their Wedding Day'. It was just fantastic and I felt so grateful to everyone who came out to support us on our big day.

The hotel we chose for the reception has changed its name a few times since we got married, but it's now called the Clanree Hotel in Letterkenny. Alcorn's had done another fabulous job and there were flower displays all over the place, which were stunning. We had silver candle-holders intertwined with flowers on every table and we had stuck an envelope under one chair; whoever found that envelope got to take the table-setting home as a gift.

When we arrived at the hotel there were hundreds of people standing outside waiting to get a glimpse of us, so again we spent some time shaking their hands and standing for pictures. Our wedding party had taken over the hotel completely for two days, so we knew everyone inside. The atmosphere was brilliant, but with all the photographs and meeting and greeting, everything was running late and I think it was nine o'clock at night before we sat down for the meal! Nobody seemed to mind because the atmosphere was so good and there were lots of canapés and drinks being served.

We had a delicious meal, but to honest I can't remember what it was now! All I know is that it was lovely. A friend of ours, Eileen Oglesby, or McPhillips as she is now known, made the wedding cake, which had about eight tiers. It had a little water feature in the middle of it and it was amazing. The speeches were great because my dad was a bit of a character and Daniel's brother James is hilarious, to say the least. He got up and recounted how a reporter had asked him before the wedding what it was like to have a famous brother and James had answered by saying, 'I don't know. You'd better ask Daniel'.

Daniel made a speech and, to be honest, I thought it would never end. It was beautiful and I think that he was so happy that he was finally there, he just kept thanking people. He went through the whole journey of our meeting and how happy he was that Siobhán and Michael were in his life, but that he only ever wanted to be a good friend to them as they already had a father. He has always been very respectful of Raymond in that sense. Our first dance was beautiful and we chose Anne Murray's 'Could I Have This Dance for The Rest Of My Life' and I floated around the dance floor. Daniel is a brilliant dancer and he has taught me, too. I love dancing with him, but I find it really hard to dance with other people. It's like he takes control and all I have to do is follow. I think we got to bed the next morning at about seven a.m. I can truly say it was one of the best days of my life.

Chapter 8

A New Life

After Daniel and I got married, we set up our home in Donegal in a place called Cruit Island, a small island which is close to Kincasslagh, and joined to the mainland by a bridge. I had been living outside Ireland for twenty-two years and it was so nice to be back home again, albeit in a different part of the country. I found the people of Donegal to be very friendly and welcoming. I have settled very well there and although I will always be a 'blow-in', I now consider it my home.

I think Donegal is one of the most beautiful counties in Ireland. It is very unspoilt with a wild natural beauty and wonderful big beaches. I think most tourists visiting Ireland nearly always opt to visit places like Kerry and the southernmost tip of the island. That probably goes back to the days of the troubles in the North, when people were afraid to travel around this area. I can assure people that Donegal is well worth the effort to travel to. And it is an effort! There are no railway links and no motorways, but we do have a small airport very near our home called Carrickfinn Airport and I can tell you that we are very glad to have it, especially with all the travelling we do. It only takes forty minutes to fly from Dublin to Donegal, but it takes about four hours to drive and the last hour of the journey is on winding and narrow roads – although they are improving all the time. We now live in a place called Meenbanad, which is only about three kilometres from Kincasslagh and five from Cruit Island.

Many people want to know what Daniel is really like and I find it very hard to put it into words without sounding completely biased. I can honestly say that I have never met anyone like him in my life before. He is the most selfless person I know and his main focus in life is trying to make other people happy in whatever way he can. That can be very frustrating at times to us lesser mortals! That's not to say that he doesn't annoy the hell out of me sometimes, but usually that's down to my lack of patience. He, on the other hand, has 'the patience of a saint', as they say. We have been together now for fourteen years and I have never once heard him refuse to have a picture taken or to sign an autograph for anyone regardless of where we are or what we are doing.

I remember one evening in particular, shortly after we were married, when we went out to a dance with some friends. Everyone was on the dance floor and Daniel and I were sitting talking in a corner. A lady came over and, without acknowledging me, asked Daniel to dance. I was really affronted, but I said nothing because I didn't want to upset anyone. Of course, Daniel agreed but, when he came back, I told him that I was really upset at what I felt to be her rudeness. His view was quite different and, I have to say, I felt a bit bad when he explained to me that the woman had probably spent some time getting herself worked up to ask him to dance and that she was probably really nervous and he would never refuse someone in that situation. He said that sometimes people don't realize how they come across when they are nervous and they do and say odd things that they wouldn't normally. He was right, of course. I have learned a lot from Daniel in this respect and he has definitely helped me to be a more tolerant person.

Having said all that, it can be really frustrating when your partner is so understanding. It can make you feel like a horrible person at times. Another example of his thought-fulness was when we were leaving Donegal to go to America after our wedding day. On the way to Dublin, Daniel asked if I would mind him taking a detour of about twenty kilometres so that he could visit a lady he knew who was sick. I was surprised that something like that would even enter his head on our way to our honeymoon, but that's Daniel for you! I was eager to get to the airport and I suppose I just wanted to be in our private bubble for a little longer, so I was a bit peeved with him.

We arrived at this small house and Daniel asked me if I would go in with him. When the lady answered the door, her face was a picture! We sat with her for about fifteen minutes and she was a lovely person. She couldn't believe that we would visit her, especially the day after our wedding and she was completely elated. When we left that house, I felt like such a selfish person: I would have been perfectly happy if we had carried on to the airport, not understand-ing that if I had, I would have denied that lady the happiness that she took from that fifteen-minute visit. It really took nothing out of me and yet it brought her such joy and happiness. I've learned not to be so selfish and whenever Daniel suggests a visit now, I never disagree.

Another time that Daniel's selflessness amazed me was

when Sir Cliff Richard came to one of his concerts. I can say without any doubt that Cliff has become a very good close friend of ours. We got to know him after he visited Donegal to attend a festival that was held in Kincasslagh every year called The Donegal Shore Festival. It was organized by Kathleen, Daniel's sister, and her husband John, along with a committee and they had a lot of help from the neighbours and the community. It was for all of Daniel's fans and they travelled from all over Ireland and the UK and from even as far as New Zealand, Australia, America and Canada to come and see where he was from. During the festival there would be lots of events organized and Daniel would do a concert on one of the nights. The main event was the ball, which was held at the end of the festival. Every year, a guest, normally a woman, would be invited, known as the 'Belle'. Daniel would never know who the guest was, so they would be brought onto the stage to surprise him. People like Gloria Hunniford, Dana, Liz Dawn from *Coronation Street*, Michelle Collins and Loretta Lynn to name but a few, have been Donegal Shore Belles. I was not in his life for the majority of these festivals, but when we became a couple, they decided to stop having a 'Belle' as he had finally found his! But they still liked to have a special guest.

For the very last ball, Kathleen wanted to have someone

really special, so she approached Sir Cliff Richard's management to see if he would be willing to attend. When he said yes, we were absolutely delighted. Sir Cliff Richard in Kincasslagh, Co. Donegal! Daniel is a huge fan of Cliff's, so I knew he would be over the moon – he was always worried that the belle wouldn't be recognized by the fans and that there would be a poor reaction when he/she walked on stage. Kathleen had told me it was Cliff, but nobody else knew. It was top secret.

Daniel asked me if the belle was well known and I said, 'Ah, yeah, people should know them.' I couldn't say if it was a man or a woman. I was bursting inside to tell him, but I just couldn't spoil the surprise. Because Cliff was staying at our house the night of the festival, Daniel was asked to go and stay at his mum's for the day. Cliff was arriving in the afternoon and we didn't want Daniel to know. I was at the house waiting for him to arrive and thinking to myself, Sir Cliff Richard is coming to stay with us. I couldn't get my head around it. Having said that, famous people don't really faze me at all. I really believe that we are all the same, regardless of what possessions or wealth we may have.

Kathleen was at the house with me when he arrived and when I opened the door, she couldn't speak. She was completely star struck! I just introduced myself and welcomed him in. I showed him his room and where the kitchen was and I told him that my house was his house and to make himself feel at home. I showed him where everything was so that he could make himself tea or coffee or whatever he wanted. I don't like to fuss over people and I don't think he would have liked being fussed over either. We had lunch and chatted away very easily.

When the night came, Daniel had to walk to one side of the stage and to turn his back and Cliff was brought out on the other side. The crowd went absolutely mad, but Daniel still had no idea who it was. Normally, he would then be asked to turn around and met his belle, but this time Cliff had his guitar with him and he just started singing: 'Got myself a cryin', talkin', sleepin', walkin', livin' doll ...' Daniel jumped around and he couldn't believe his eyes.

It was a great night and Cliff stayed with us in our home on Cruit Island, so we got to know him fairly well. Daniel had met him on a few occasions prior to that, but only in a professional capacity. We got on so well with him during the festival because he's a charming and funny man and since then we have met up fairly regularly and had many holidays together. Cliff has a gentle soul and I have never heard him say a bad word about anyone. Actually, Daniel and Cliff have a lot of similarities.

Which brings me back to why Daniel's selflessness amazes me. Before Daniel really got to know Cliff, he was a huge fan. He had always admired him and his music and he had recorded some of his songs, so for him to get to know Cliff on a personal level was a real privilege. However, Daniel is still Daniel! One time, shortly after we became friends, he was in concert near London and Cliff decided that he would come to see him perform. Cliff had never been before, so when he told Daniel he was coming, Daniel was really excited. We arranged to have dinner straight after the show in a private room in the theatre. Cliff was with Gloria Hunniford and her husband, Stephen, and a few friends whom we also knew.

As many of Daniel's fans will know, he takes time with anyone that wants to stay after the concert and meet him. He has always done it and I guess he always will. On this occasion, though, I suggested to him that, as I had arranged dinner with Cliff straight after the show, maybe he could explain to the audience that he couldn't meet them that night and why. I was sure that, as fans, they would understand what it might be like to have dinner with your idol!

Daniel was adamant that he just couldn't do that to his fans. He said he would be really quick and would join us as soon as he could. I took him at his word because I know how important this dinner was to him. Unfortunately, as Daniel stayed until the last fan had left, which was about two hours later, dinner was well finished and Cliff was just about to leave. All Daniel got to do was have a picture and say goodbye. How many other people would turn down the chance to have dinner with their idol so that their fans could say hello and have a picture taken with him? It wasn't even as though he was cutting the concert short! I felt very sorry for him, but I really admired his principles that night. He felt that his fans had travelled from all over the place just to see and meet him and he couldn't deny them. That's why he has such a loyal following.

The Daniel that I know around the house is fairly quiet. He is very undemanding and doesn't ask for much. He's very easy to live with and always even-tempered. He's one of those people who wakes up in the morning with a big smile on his face. I, on the other hand, am the complete opposite and it takes me a good half an hour before I can even be approached by another human being! He also gets stuck in with the cleaning, washing and vacuuming and the only thing he doesn't really do is cook. When it comes to food, he has very simple tastes. I suppose you could say that Daniel eats to be fed, but not for the enjoyment of it. On the other hand, I love food and wine and for me there is nothing better than a really nice meal with a good bottle of wine and some interesting conversation.

I have to say, Daniel is getting more adventurous with his food because I like to get him to try new things when I can. He never really gets hungry, which I find very strange. If I don't eat regularly I get very narky and usually end up with a headache, but Daniel could go all day and only realize at night that he hasn't eaten. He doesn't really drink apart from the odd glass of champagne or Baileys Irish Cream liqueur on a special occasion. I have seen him drink more than that on no more than a couple of times since I've known him, and he was no different with the drink than he was without it. Unfortunately, the next day, he suffered terribly, so it really wasn't worth his while. Drink just doesn't suit him. Anyway, Daniel doesn't need drink to enjoy himself. He is very lucky in that respect. When we are in Tenerife, we go to the music pubs from time to time and he never gets bored or wants to leave, even when there are drunk people around him. When I have no drink taken, I find drunk people really irritating! He seems to enjoy the *craic* as he is and I say, 'Good for him.' The plus side for me is that I drive to the pub and he drives home! What better arrangement could a woman have? I have to be honest and say that an odd time I would love to be able to share a nice bottle of wine with him but, overall, I prefer the fact that he is a non-drinker.

I dread to think what my life would be like without Daniel. It's not that I am afraid of being alone, but now that I have found someone that I am so connected to, I really wouldn't want to lose that. Daniel has the ability to calm me and to make me feel safe. I feel that he adds so much to my life as a person. I love knowing that he is out there, wherever that may be and that he's caring about me. That's a wonderful feeling and what I missed most when I was single. We have very separate lives at times. I enjoy having my own space to do the things that I want to do, but I always know that there is someone there who is interested in my well-being.

We usually talk at least twice a day on Skype when he is touring and the fact that I can see him when we are talking makes a big difference. It never feels as if he is too far away. When we are together, it is just so easy. With the troubles I had in my first marriage, I never realized how good it could be to be with someone that you are totally comfortable with in every way. I would trust Daniel with my life.

He has also been absolutely wonderful to my children and they both love him very much. Even though their father is very active in their lives, they love Daniel and consider him to be 'Dad number two'!

Daniel has known Siobhán since she was twelve and Michael since he was ten. Daniel has always said that he never wanted to be a father to them because they have their own father: he just wanted to be the best friend he could be and he wanted them to be able to come to him if they ever needed anything. They have a great banter between them and they are very comfortable with each other. I remember when Siobhán was about fourteen she was really into Eminem, the rap singer, and she had posters of him all over her bedroom wall. Before she came home from school one time, Daniel got a load of his promotional photos and stuck them over Eminem's face on every poster. It was so funny to see her reaction. Another time, when she was about sixteen, she brought her boyfriend to Donegal for the weekend. She was a bit nervous about it and she kept reminding us not to be asking him questions and to leave them alone. Daniel very calmly and seriously asked her when she wanted him to sing for the boyfriend. Should he sing when he arrived at the front door, or should he wait until they were having dinner? As you can imagine, Siobhán was horrified and she started squealing, but I thought it was so funny.

I always thought that it was such a shame that Daniel didn't have any children of his own. When we married first, we both decided that we would try for a baby, but it never happened. I suppose it just wasn't meant to be. I felt bad for Daniel because I think parenthood is such a wonderful thing but, on reflection, it wasn't something that he wanted so badly that he would have been prepared to go to any lengths to become a father. He says now that that time has passed, he can be glad that we didn't have a baby because our lives would be very different. He's right, of course, and quite honestly, I know that I don't have the energy that I once had either. I know that he is as happy as he can be with the way things turned out and that he has the freedom to do as he pleases with his time off.

Daniel will be very embarrassed when he reads this chapter of the book, as he is very uncomfortable with anyone praising him. This time he is just going to have to put up with it: it's my story after all! I am so blessed and privileged that such a unique human being asked me to be part of his life and for that I am thankful every day. It's true though, that my life with Daniel is so very different to the life I had before I met him. I feel a little bit like Cinderella. Before I met him I was on my own and certainly missing that special someone in my life. I worked hard to pay my bills and to keep my head above water, as most of us have to do. I had a failed marriage behind me and I had suffered depression in varying degrees. I really didn't know where my life was headed and I didn't like that feeling. Tenerife was a complete break from everything for me. A real chance to get away from it all and to focus on what I wanted out of life. Never in a million years did I think when I went there that I would end up marrying a handsome single millionaire – because that's what he was! That's what I mean when I say I felt like Cinderella: not that I was waiting for Prince Charming because I had learned to live my life on my own terms, but because my life has changed completely in every respect since then.

I noticed a number of changes, once Daniel and I were married. Things were suddenly very different for me. For a start, I didn't work because I wouldn't have been able to have a job and just take off whenever Daniel was home, otherwise I would never see him, but I was a very independent person before I met Daniel. After we married, it was really strange not having my own money. I found it hard relying on him for everything. Daniel is very generous and would never deny me anything, but that was not the point. I missed having my own wages and I missed the satisfaction that I got from working. I don't want to sound like I'm complaining because I'm not! It was just a strange position to be in.

After a few years of not working, I began to feel like I had no purpose in life because I had nothing to keep me stimulated and nothing to give me a sense of achievement. That's very important in life for your self-respect. That's when I sat down with Jack Black and set some goals for myself, such as my goal to set up a mental health charity in Donegal and to take more time for exercise. Since then I have felt much more fulfilled because I have something worthwhile to aim for. It has given me a purpose.

I have gotten used to being a 'kept' woman, but I still like to earn my own wee bit of money and to contribute to the household when I can. I don't like to waste money. When I go shopping for clothes, I still automatically head for the sale or bargain rail, even though I don't need to. I suppose we all put different values on things. For example, my daughter just loves designer handbags. She was always telling me to buy a Louis Vuitton bag and that it was an investment. I like handbags, but I don't see the necessity of paying hundreds of euro for one just because it has a designer label on it. However, I took her advice and I did buy a Vuitton 'Bucket' bag because it would look good and last me for ever. It never gave me a thrill having it, but every time I saw Siobhán she would tell me how gorgeous the bag was. In the end, I gave it to her because I had no regard for it and I knew that she would get far more pleasure from it than I did.

To me, bags, jewellery and designer clothes are lovely things to have, but they are only 'things'. I don't need them to live a worthwhile life, so I'm not bothered if I have them or not. I don't disagree with people wanting these things and I do have some designer clothes in my wardrobe, which is lovely, but they don't define me as a person. We are all different and different things push our buttons.

Make-up is another thing that I can take or leave. It's great to put on every now and then when I'm going some-where nice, but I certainly don't wear it all the time. I find it a real pain having to put it on and then take it all off when I'm going to bed. I'm aware that I have 'something' on my face and I can't wait to take it off and feel that clean, fresh feeling again. Obviously, I have to wear it a lot more often since I met Daniel because of the amount of functions we have to attend. I want to look nice for myself and for Daniel. I don't want people looking at me and saying, 'What on earth is he doing with her? Look at the state of her'! So I try my best to look as good as I can when I need to – that's why I did that make-up course that I mentioned at the beginning of the book – to make it as easy for myself as possible. It was money well spent and I'm very glad I did it. Friends used to ask me if I had someone to do my hair and make-up all the time, but that's just fantasy. I don't have someone telling me what to wear and it certainly shows sometimes! I wish I had. Life is pretty normal most of the time, but if I am doing something on TV I will sometimes hire a make-up artist so that I don't have to worry about that side of things. That doesn't happen very often though.

The other thing I have noticed since being married to Daniel is that people seem to look at me in a different way. I am just the same person I always have been, but in other people's eyes, I am perceived as someone who is special, I suppose. When you are with someone very well known, people think that your life is privileged. It is, to some extent, because you get to see and meet people whom you would never normally meet and you get to go places that you wouldn't normally go. And, of course, it is wonderful not to have to worry about paying your bills, but everything in life is relative. Nobody's life is perfect. You still have your worries and your ups and downs. You still have health issues, as I have discovered. As they say, 'your health is your wealth' and I know that only too well. No matter what the circumstances, you are still just a human being trying to make the best of your life.

I have been to some wonderful events in London as a guest of Sir Cliff and I would find myself in a room full of very wealthy people, celebrities and stars, and wonder to myself how I ever got there. Me, Majella Roche from Thurles in Co. Tipperary! Gloria Hunniford has become a good friend, too, and has been very supportive during my cancer experience. I have met Cilla Black many times and I found her to be full of humour. There are lots of people like that whom I have met, but that doesn't really matter. All I see is the person. Some of them are lovely and others are very shallow. That's life. I am not easily impressed by celebrity. As I have said before, we are all the same in this world and having more money or fame does not make a better person. That comes from within.

People think that being recognized when we are out must be very annoying, but really it's not at all. Generally the public are very nice and it takes nothing out of me to say hello to someone. When people do approach us, it is usually to say that they are thinking of us or praying for us or whatever. That's a nice thing. That's a privilege.

One thing I love about my new life is Donegal. I love the outdoors and I love to spend the summer outside as much as I can when the weather permits. I also love the water and being near it and I spend a lot of time in the summer months on a little island off the coast called Owey Island. It's where Daniel's mother was born and raised and it's a wonderfully peaceful place to be. There are a few houses on it, which have been renovated over the past few years and people go out there for weekends and holidays to get away from it all. Just like in Julia's time, there is no electricity, running water or roads on the island. When night time falls, it gets completely dark because there are no street lights and the stars look absolutely wonderful. Self-sufficiency is the aim as much as possible and it's a great feeling to know that you don't need all the modern conveniences to live a simple life. I am not saying that I don't want them, but when I stay on the island, I find it very liberating to know that I can survive on very little for those few weeks and still have a wonderful time.

Chapter 9

My Cancer Journey

In July 2013, I was visiting friends in London. I was lying on the bed one very warm afternoon, reading a book, when I scratched my left breast. I felt straight away that there was a small lump close to the nipple. I really wasn't very concerned as I'd had about four lumps in my breasts over the years. The first one was removed when I was only twenty-one. The others were all examined by my GP and a fine-needle aspiration was performed immediately. Each time a cyst was diagnosed and no further treatment was necessary. I believe that nowadays you are routinely sent to a breast clinic for assessment.

I decided to call my GP straight away to make an appointment to have the lump assessed as I never take these things for granted. Although I didn't expect the worst, while I was waiting for my appointment the following week, part of me wondered, 'What if?' I suppose your mind wanders and you think of all sorts of scenarios, but I kept myself in check and when I began to worry, would tell myself not to be a drama queen, expecting the worst. I knew that in all likelihood, it was a cyst yet again: I would have been far more surprised at a cancer diagnosis.

The appointment was made by my GP for the Beacon Hospital in Sandyford, Dublin. Daniel came with me on the day and I would say he was probably more worried than I was. First we went into the consultant's office and met Mr Terry Boyle, Consultant Breast Surgeon at the Beacon. He explained to me that all patients who presented with breast lumps underwent a triple assessment, which would include an examination, scan and biopsy, if that was deemed necessary. He examined me and told me that he wasn't very concerned about my lump, but that he would send me for a mammogram just to be on the safe side. The mammogram wasn't very clear, so I was then sent for an ultrasound. As I was lying there looking at the screen, I could see some black holes, which I presumed were cysts, and I felt quite relieved as I was sure there was nothing untoward. The radiographer then said that she wanted to do a needle biopsy of the tissue. I presumed that this was like the fine-needle aspiration, where she would take out the fluid just to analyse it. Obviously, she had seen something that I hadn't. I then went back to Mr Boyle's office and he told me that the results would be in the following Thursday evening and that they would call me as soon as they were available.

I went up to Donegal as my mother and father were staying with me for a few days and there's no place nicer in the summer time. I didn't really think about it during those few days as I was busy pottering about with Mum and Dad. Early on Thursday afternoon my phone rang and it was the breast-care nurse from the Beacon Hospital. She told me that the tests were inconclusive and that they needed to see me again. I didn't really understand what she meant, and even though she told me that I didn't need to come to Dublin until Monday, I was keen to get it sorted straight away, so I told her I would be down on Friday morning. She asked me if I would be travelling alone to Dublin and when I asked her why, she explained to me that as it was such a long journey, it would be nice if I had company on the way. I wasn't sure whether she was being completely open with me and part of me wondered if this was to protect me in some way, but as I'm a positive thinker nowadays, I decided that it was just my imagination again.

Daniel had gone to Tenerife a couple of days earlier as we were pretty sure that everything was going to be fine. He had signed up for a Spanish course and he was doing some golfing with a couple of his friends. When I phoned him to tell him that I had to go back to Dublin, he immediately said he was going to fly home. I told him not to be ridiculous and that he should stay for the week as planned. 'You're overreacting,' I told him. He was insistent and he managed to get a flight that evening. I didn't want to worry Mum and Dad, so I told them that there was nothing to worry about: the hospital just needed to do one of the tests again. They seemed happy enough with that, which was a relief.

As I drove down to Dublin that evening, all sorts of things started running through my brain and I had to stop myself from being overwhelmed by negative thoughts. I believe there is no point in worrying about something until you have all the information. You could spend all your time thinking 'what if' and then find out that you're anxious about nothing. I thought, what was the point of getting myself into a state when I didn't know for sure what the facts were but, even so, I found it hard to shake the thought that something might be wrong.

The next day, Daniel and I returned to the Beacon Hospital and checked in at reception. I was very surprised that there were no other people in the waiting area. The previous time I'd been there it had been very busy and there were a lot of women waiting to be seen. The receptionist told us that Mr Boyle would be late and suggested we go for a coffee while we were waiting. Again, I was surprised because I hadn't been expecting to meet the consultant: after all, I only needed one of the tests to be done again. Why would Terry, as I had started to refer to him then, need to be there to have that done? Now I really was beginning to get worried.

We went back to reception after about an hour and Terry called us into his office. Daniel and I sat next to each other and we held hands as he opened my file. I will always remember that first sentence: 'You are Majella O'Donnell and you presented yourself to this clinic with a lump in your left breast. You underwent the triple assessment and had a biopsy taken of your breast tissue. The biopsy has shown that there are cancerous cells present in your breast.' He wasn't looking at me when he read from the file, but I never found Terry to be cold or uncaring. He was reading the file and, I suppose, trying not to sound alarmist. A person in his line of work must have to deliver this kind of news lots of times every day. Not only do you have to be a good surgeon and know about your patient, but you also have to have the skills to deliver news like that to very different types of people. How do you know what the right way is? Is the right way the same for every patient? I doubt it. I wanted the truth, with no fluffiness. I didn't want to be sheltered in any way. Just tell me the facts and let me deal with it in whatever way I have to, that was my thinking. As far as I was concerned, Terry's delivery of my cancer diagnosis was spot on for me. It must be a terrible part of any consultant's job when they have to deliver bad news to a patient. I knew he was trying to be as gentle as he could.

When he'd finished, I just said: 'So ... What does that mean?' It was silly, really, because I knew exactly what it meant, but I suppose what I should have said was, 'How bad is it and where do we go from here?' At that moment, Daniel squeezed my hand and I could see tears in his eyes. I knew that he was waiting for my reaction to see how I was handling it: if I fell apart, then he probably would, too, but I didn't feel panicked or tearful, for some reason. I can't explain it, but it was as if it wasn't really happening to me. It didn't seem like a shock because Terry had never said, 'You have cancer'. He'd just said there were cancerous cells present. Those words didn't seem to hit my brain as hard and, for that, I will always be thankful to Terry.

He then went on to explain that I was lucky in that I had

caught it very early and it was very small, just under 2 centimetres. He told me they would do an MRI scan to see if the cancer had spread anywhere else. That was done immediately and I also had various blood tests that day. When I was finished with all the tests, I went back to meet Terry and he told me that there were no signs of the cancer having spread to any other parts of my body. I was so glad to hear that as I had visions of it being all around my body at that stage. The next procedure would be a lumpectomy, which would be carried out as soon as possible. I know that I surprised him when I told him that I wanted a mastectomy straight away. Previously when I had found lumps in my breast, I had always said that if they turned out to be cancerous, I would have a mastectomy, no question. I just felt that my chances of the cancer returning would be far less if my breast was removed. I had had a couple of friends who'd had breast cancer and mastectomies and they looked fantastic, so I wasn't concerned about the outcome cosmetically.

Terry listened to what I had to say, but told me that it would be far better to have the lumpectomy first and then decide on what course of action to take, once we knew what type of cancer we were dealing with. I struggled with that and I felt that he was trying to put me off having the mastectomy. I made him promise me that if I had the lumpectomy, I could then have the mastectomy afterwards.

I have to say that it took him a good two weeks to convince me to do the lumpectomy first, but I am very glad that he did. He explained that until they had taken out the lump and assessed it, they didn't really know what they were dealing with and if I went ahead and insisted on a mastectomy first, it could be detrimental to the treatment afterwards. If I had problems healing after the mastectomy or I developed any infections because of it, I might not be able to get my treatment for a long time and that could be very risky. I suppose I just thought that if I had a mastectomy, I could deal with the whole thing very quickly and matter of factly and that would be it. That is so me! Just deal with it, get on and don't look back. I had to learn to be patient and to deal with one thing at a time.

So, that was it. I had breast cancer and I now had to go home and face what all of that meant for me. I had no idea where to start. Firstly, I had to let it sink in myself. I couldn't believe that I had cancer in me. I felt fine and looked fine, but I had been told it, so it was true. Then I started to think about who I had to tell. I was shocked, so I knew that everyone else would be too. I concentrated on my family and I let Daniel tell our friends. I wondered how on earth I was going to deal with Siobhán and Michael.

Before I left the hospital that day, one of the breast-care nurses took me into a room to see if I wanted to ask any questions. I couldn't think straight and the only thing I asked her was, 'Do I have to pay for my car parking today as I've been here for five hours?' Where on earth did that come from? I suppose that I was still trying to take it all in. Thankfully the breast-care nurses are really nice and very helpful and are on hand to answer any questions you have whenever you have them. They try to support you all the way through the process of the cancer journey and, for me, they were wonderful.

When we left the clinic, I had to phone Mum and Dad as they were waiting on news from me and I knew they'd worry. I also knew that I couldn't tell them the truth over the phone, so I had to lie. That is something that I very rarely do, so I felt very uncomfortable about it, but I knew that it would be better to talk to them in person. I took a deep breath and phoned and my Mum said, 'Well, what's happened'?

'Everything's fine,' I said.

'Oh, that's great news. We were very worried there for a while.'

I tried to get off the phone as quickly as possible so that she wouldn't sense that anything was wrong.

Daniel and I flew back to Donegal that evening where I had to face my parents and tell them the news that I'm sure no parent wants to hear: that their child has cancer.

We knew that it would be best to talk to them sitting down all together, so when we got up to Donegal we decided to play a game of cards, so we all sat down at the table. That was the only way I could face them without them panicking. As Daniel dealt the cards, I reached my hands across the table and caught each of Mum's and Dad's hands in mine and I said: 'I'm sorry, but I wasn't telling you the truth when I called you. I'm afraid I have breast cancer.' Dad immediately said to Mum, 'I told you she might be lying to us!' I then explained that they had caught it early and that my prognosis was very good, which seemed to calm them a little. I believe that people take their cue from whomever is delivering bad news and if you deliver it in as positive a way as possible, it does help to soften the blow. Of course, they were worried sick, but if I had told them whilst bawling and crying then they would have been far more upset. Anyway, I didn't feel like that. I didn't feel upset or sad. I didn't feel that I had cancer, so it was all a bit unreal saying the words. I said them, but I didn't really believe them, I suppose.

My mother was very quiet, which surprised me and she didn't cry or say much. I hadn't seen my mother in those circumstances before and I thought she would react differently. I thought she would be inconsolable, but that was not the case. She was very much in control, but since my father's sudden death, I realize that that's how my mum copes with shock. She just goes quiet and retreats into herself. I explained everything about my diagnosis and the treatment as best I could and was very matter of fact about the whole thing. I think when they saw that I felt quite strong, it helped them to cope better. And at that point, I did feel strong. I had no reason to believe that I couldn't fight and win this battle and I'm always up for a challenge.

However, that night when I went to bed, all I could think about was telling my children. How on earth was I going to break the news that their mother had cancer? I knew that if I had heard that about my mother, I would've been distraught. They would probably think that I was going to die. I really didn't want to frighten them and I wanted to give them as many facts as I could at same time, so I decided to meet them in person to explain the news to them in detail. Siobhán and Michael were both working and living in London at the time, so Daniel and I decided that we would travel to meet them so that I could explain everything face-to-face. We organized to see them the following week and I had to keep the news of my cancer quiet because I was afraid they would hear it from somebody else in the family. I had told my mum and dad and my sisters and brother. Daniel told his sisters and brothers, so there was always a possibility that someone might say something and be overheard or whatever. You know how things can get out so quickly nowadays with Facebook and Twitter. I didn't want that to happen. As I lay in bed with all these thoughts going through my head, I got very frightened and I started to cry. Daniel put his arms around me and held me and said nothing. There was nothing he could say and I was glad that he realized that that was all I needed at that time. I just needed him to put his arms around me and to know that he was there for me if I needed him. That was the only time that I cried about being diagnosed with cancer, the only time that I allowed myself to give in to feeling sorry for myself. I knew that from then on, I needed to be strong if I was to face the journey that was ahead of me.

The following week, Daniel and I travelled to London and we met Siobhán and Michael at a friend's house before we were due to go out for dinner. I was dreading the thought of telling them and I was scared of their reaction because, as a mother, I wanted to protect them from the pain I knew they were going to feel. I sat between them on the settee and explained to them that I had something to tell them. Then I just couldn't speak. The words just wouldn't come out. I could feel the tears starting to well up inside me and thankfully Daniel realized what was happening and he told them. Once he had said the word 'cancer', I was fine and I was able to pick up the story and tell them that I was going to be all right.

Once again, I was surprised by their reaction. I expected them to start screaming and crying, but there was none of that. They were both very calm, but I could see a great sadness in their eyes. I think when they saw that I wasn't frightened and that the treatment was very successful nowadays, they were much less fearful then they might have been. I think it's a lack of knowledge that creates fear and, once I explained a bit about what was happening, they were much more relaxed. Of course, there were a few tears, but only tears of sadness, not hysterical tears as I had expected. I was so glad when that was over. I had been worrying for three days about how they would react and they took it so much better than I could have imagined.

Daniel and I then started to discuss how we would handle the situation over the next few months. He had a lot of tours in his diary and straight away he said he would cancel everything for the foreseeable future. I really didn't want him to do that. To me, it was far too drastic. I wanted things to go on as normally as possible under the circumstances. I am the type of person who doesn't like to be fussed over when I am sick. I also knew that this was a battle I had to undertake on my own and only I could do it. I needed to know that Daniel was there for me if I needed him, but I didn't want him to be sitting around waiting on me hand and foot. I had a few engagements in my own diary that I needed to cancel and I felt very bad about doing so. I knew that I was letting people down at the last minute and that is not my style.

Once we had told both our families, we decided that it would be easier to make a public announcement about my cancer so that people could understand our reasons for cancelling things in the following months.

In the past, I have spoken about my experience with depression and cancer to me was no different. It is something that many people face in all walks of life every single day. As I was open about my depression, I wanted to be open about cancer, too. As far as I'm concerned, we are all on this earth together and regardless of our colour, creed, nationality or culture we all face similar tribulations in life. We all have to get on and get through difficult situations as best as we can. If we can help each other in doing so then I am happy to do my part. I wanted to tell people how it was and then to just get on with dealing with it.

Depression wasn't something that I dwelt on or that defined me in any way. I spoke about it quite by accident really. I was being interviewed by Ryan Tubridy on his radio show just about my life in general and, I suppose, life since meeting Daniel. I was talking about all sorts of things and I mentioned that I had suffered from bouts of depression. Ryan picked up on this straight away and delved a bit deeper, asking me all sorts of questions about it, which I had no problem answering. The next day, the newspapers reported that I had 'come out' about suffering from this illness and how brave I was to be open about it. The truth is, I was never 'in', as far as I was concerned. You see, I didn't see it as a big deal. It was a part of my life and that's all. I am not ashamed about it, therefore I have no need to hide it. I am only human and none of us is perfect, so why should I feel bad or try to hide it. Other people have blood pressure or diabetes and they're not afraid to admit that. The reaction surprised me because I didn't make a conscious decision to talk about it to Ryan, it was just part of my story.

A couple of weeks later, I had the lumpectomy and I was then diagnosed with invasive ductal carcinoma. This is the most common form of breast cancer and therefore it has a very high chance of a cure if found early. I also had some of my lymph nodes removed and they showed that there were microscopic cancer cells present. A small amount of the breast-cancer tissue was also sent to America for an Oncotype DX test. This test looks at the activity of a group of twenty-one genes in your tumour and can help to give more information about your cancer. This helps doctors to decide if you will benefit from chemotherapy as part of your treatment. The test is only helpful for patients with certain types of breast cancer and in the early stages. My cancer was oestrogen-receptor positive, which means that it was stimulated by the hormone oestrogen and was suitable for the test. The test also gives an indication of the likelihood of recurrence of the cancer and my result showed that I had an intermediate chance of recurrence. I suppose that means I have about a twenty per cent chance of it returning in the future.

Once the operation was over, I met my oncologist, Dr Jennifer Westrup, Consultant Medical Oncologist at the Beacon Hospital, to discuss what course of treatment was best for me. Having seen my results, she recommended that I have a course of chemotherapy to reduce the possibility of my cancer returning. Radiation treats the area where the cancer has been found, but chemotherapy treats the whole body, in case any rogue cancer cells have travelled to a different part of the body. It literally kills any new cells, whether they are good or bad cells, from the top of your head to the tips of your toes. Jenny, as she asked me to call her, also advised that I should have six-and-a-half weeks of radiation to the affected breast once my chemotherapy was finished. She told me that, once I had completed chemotherapy and radiation, I would be on hormonal therapy for the following five years.

When Jenny told me that I would have to have chemotherapy, I was absolutely shocked, more shocked then when I had been told that I had cancer. You see, I presumed that I would have a lumpectomy, followed by radiation and then the hormone treatment and that would be it. Having to have chemotherapy was serious stuff and I certainly didn't think that my cancer was that serious. I also knew that I was going to lose my hair and this would really bring home to me that I did in fact have the big 'C' as it is sometimes called. It still didn't feel real to me, but as I was going to lose my hair, there was no way I could avoid the reality of it. I was going to be sick, too. With a lumpectomy and radiation, there is no sickness or nausea, so that didn't frighten me. However, chemotherapy was another thing altogether. All I had seen of chemotherapy before was people going bald, looking really pale, losing a lot of weight and vomiting a lot. That really frightened me and that's why I was so shocked that I had to have that treatment. Up until then, I didn't feel sick, but I knew that to fight this disease I would have to put my body through a very gruelling few months to make myself better.

When I thought about the effects of the chemo, I wondered what it would be like to have my hair coming out of my head in handfuls. I didn't like that idea at all. When I had seen cancer patients on TV programmes or films brushing their hair and loads of it coming out, it made me feel a bit sick, but I knew that I could never go through that. In the end, most people shave their heads anyway because sometimes it doesn't fall out evenly and you have bald patches all over your head. To me, that was a terrifying thought.

I was determined that life would go on as normally as possible, even though I was having chemotherapy. Daniel and I had booked a week's holiday in Rome in late September, before I'd got the news, so when we were planning the start date for the chemo, we tried to work it around that holiday so that I would still be able to go. I really wanted things to be as normal as possible. My first chemo date was Thursday 12 September and I was due to go away on 23 September. That would give me a full week to get over the effects of the drugs and I decided that if I didn't feel up to it then, I wouldn't go.

I had to wait for at least three weeks after the lumpectomy surgery, which I had had on Friday 26 July, before chemotherapy could start. I didn't feel too bad during that time because at least I knew I was dealing with things. The lumpectomy was over, I knew what type of cancer I was dealing with and my chemotherapy was starting in three weeks. I was actually eager for the twelfth to arrive because I just wanted to get on with it. I felt that the sooner I started the treatment, the sooner it would be over.

My mother had come to stay with me in Dublin for the whole time I was having chemo, but we never really talked about the cancer as such, only about how I was feeling each day. She got to see the pattern, so she knew when I was starting to feel well again after chemo. I thought there was no point dwelling on the cancer. For me, the least energy I could give it the better. Not because I needed the energy myself, but because if I was thinking about it constantly, I would be fuelling it with my energy. I was dealing with it the best way possible, so it was just a case of getting on with it. It was great to have Mum there, because I knew that if I needed anything, all I had to do was ask. She would cook whatever I fancied and if I didn't want to eat or talk she would understand and leave me alone. My mum is wonderful in that respect.

I arrived at the oncology department on the morning of my chemotherapy and I felt surprisingly calm. I was just so glad to be there and to be getting the first session over with. I didn't really know what to expect, but it really wasn't that bad at all. The room had about fifteen large comfortable chairs all set a few feet apart from each other. I was told I could take any seat I wanted and I was asked if I would like any tea or coffee. The nurse came to insert a cannula in my arm through which the drugs would be administered. She explained what would happen and told me that if I felt in anyway uncomfortable, light-headed or sick, to tell her immediately. First they give you anti-sickness drugs through the cannula and then they give you the chemotherapy treatment, which has been specially made up for each individual. I kept wondering if I would feel the chemotherapy going through me, but I didn't feel anything unusual at all. It was like having a saline drip in my arm. I had my iPad with me and I Skyped Daniel because I wanted him to see that everything was fine and that I was okay. I had a cup of tea and sandwich while I was having the chemo and I have to say that the whole process was very straightforward and not in the slightest bit uncomfortable.

I was delighted with myself at this stage, partly because I knew one session was over and partly because I was on steroids and they were giving me a false sense of wellbeing. I was having my head shaved the next evening on *The Late Late Show* and I was really hoping that I would stay feeling as good as I was feeling, at least until that was over. Friday came and, thankfully, I still felt pretty good. As you know, I did the show and I was very glad when it was all over and it had received such a wonderful response from the public: more importantly, that I'd raised so much money for charity.

On Saturday morning I still felt okay and the whole day was taken up with calls and messages from well-wishers about the head shave the previous night. However, by the time Sunday arrived, I had finished my course of steroids and I was starting to feel pretty bad. On Monday morning, when Ryan Tubridy called me on live radio to see how I was doing, I was hardly able to speak, but I wanted to go on to thank everybody for their generosity over the weekend. As I said at the beginning of the book, I was absolutely amazed and shocked when Ryan told me that the Irish Cancer Society had received €250,000 up to that point. I just couldn't believe it. Friends of mine had told me that everybody was talking about it and that so many people were still continuing to pledge money on the society's website. I could feel the tears in my eyes and I had a lump in my throat. I was so happy that I had made the decision to shave my hair off. It had all been worthwhile.

As the day progressed, I felt weaker and weaker and all I could do was stay in bed and try to sleep it off. Tuesday was a bad day and I have to say that I find it very difficult to put into words exactly what it felt like. Of course, I felt extremely tired, but that wasn't the worst thing. I felt like the drugs were messing with my brain. I couldn't think straight or even have the smallest conversation with my mother. I couldn't concentrate on anything and my mind literally felt as though it was poisoned, which I suppose it was. One minute I would be lying down and then I would have to sit up or get up and move about and then I would feel that I needed to lie down again. I had weird, very vivid dreams and I would wake up feeling really unsettled. The one thing I was glad about was the fact that I didn't feel nauseous. The anti-sickness drugs are very good these days and if you take them regularly, you can avoid the nausea and vomiting. The downside to the anti-sickness drugs is that they make you constipated, which isn't very pleasant either.

By Wednesday, I was starting to feel a little bit better. My head felt a bit clearer and I didn't feel as out of control as I had done on the previous days. I was only slightly better though, and I still spent most of the day in bed, but at least I knew that things were beginning to improve. I didn't really eat very much for those three days, but when Thursday arrived, I managed to have a little piece of mashed potato with baked beans and it tasted wonderful.

When 23 September arrived, I was feeling pretty good and delighted that I was able to go to Rome as planned. I was very careful while I was away, making sure that I washed my hands regularly to avoid any infection. This is because chemotherapy kills all the new cells in your body and your immune system becomes very low and you are very susceptible to infection. I wore a mask whenever I was in crowded public places like the bus or the aeroplane. I thought I was coping pretty well.

After about three days, I was putting on some make-up in the bathroom and I rubbed my head. Hundreds and hundreds of little hairs fell into the sink and it was the strangest feeling to see that happen, especially as the hair was dark and the sink was white. I was so glad that I had shaved it because I would have hated big clumps of hair coming out. This just felt strange in a funny kind of way!

Every time I went to the sink after that, I would rub my head again to see how many more hairs would fall out. It was quite amazing to realize how many hair follicles I had in my head. I have very fine hair, like a baby's, and I always thought I didn't have much of it, but I was wrong.

We had a great week in Rome and, thankfully, I didn't pick up any infections. If I had picked one up, it might have meant that I would have had to postpone my second session of chemo and I just wanted to get the whole thing over and done with as soon as possible. A few days after I returned, I was in for my second session of chemotherapy.

As I went through each session, the pattern was pretty much the same. The first two days after chemotherapy were fine and then I would be pretty bad for the following three days, before things started to improve. I was very lucky in that I had no medical problems whatsoever during that time.

My father died very suddenly after my second session of chemotherapy and I was just so grateful that I was at the stage when I could travel, otherwise I don't know what I would've done. When I was travelling out to Tenerife, I called my oncologist to check that it was OK for me to travel. She said, 'Majella, your father is number one, but please remember that you are a very close second.' I wore a mask every time I was in public and I changed it regularly. I kept washing my hands and I tried not to have too much physical contact with my friends and family. Because the whole thing was such a shock, I think I was driven by adrenalin most of the week I was there. I tend to be the organizer in my family, or I seem to have assumed that role along the way, probably because I like things to be done efficiently and quickly so I take charge. That kept me very active and Mum kept telling me to slow down, as did Daniel and all my family, but I guess I just cope better when I'm running around organising everything. I feel that I'm doing something useful and that keeps me going. Thank God I had no setbacks at all. I think Dad looked after me in that respect.

I suppose I was lucky in that my chemo sessions went well and that I never had any medical setbacks, unlike many other people. I was also astonished at the level of public support I received during this time: hundreds and hundreds of cards and letters from people sending their best wishes and praying for me. I got huge support from so many people I didn't even know or had never met. Their kindness and generosity amazed me and really helped me on my journey. To be honest, it was very difficult for me to pray for myself when I had cancer. I felt that I didn't have the right to ask to be cured because why should I be cured above anyone else? I had been given this disease and I had to deal with it. This was my turn to carry my cross. I couldn't say 'why me?' because I knew there was no reason that it *shouldn't* be me. I believed that if I had cancer, that was the way it was meant to be. That was my path in life and I had to walk it. No amount of complaining or blaming was going to change anything. Anyway, I needed all my strength to deal with the treatment and with Dad's death, and I wasn't going to waste it on futile moaning.

When I was coming to the end of my chemotherapy sessions, I had another meeting with Mr Boyle and I told him that I still wanted to go ahead with the mastectomy. In fact, I decided that I was going to have a double mastectomy. I had thought a lot about it during the previous weeks and felt that this was the right decision for me. Maybe if I had been younger, my decision would've been different. I had my two children and I had a loving, supportive husband. I knew that my breasts were something that I could live without. When I thought about a single mastectomy, I worried about what the other breast would look like. A friend of mine who had had a single mastectomy in the past underwent various operations in a bid to make her breasts look similar. In the end, she had her second breast removed and reconstructed so that both breasts looked and felt the same. I understood that completely as I would've found it very difficult to look at two totally different breasts on my body. I felt that if I had the double mastectomy, then I would never need to worry about breast lumps in the future and they would both look and feel the same. Terry was happy that I had given it a lot of thought and that I had researched the options and was realistic about the results and he made an appointment with Mr Peter Meagher, a plastic and reconstruction surgeon at the Beacon Hospital. We discussed my expectations and what the operation would involve and we set a date of 14 February for the surgery. This meant that I had about two months from the end of my chemotherapy to the operation when I could relax and get myself strong again. That was a much-needed break and Daniel and I spent it in Tenerife. Daniel was heading to Australia and New Zealand in February to go on tour. I was happy that we had the time together in January and that he would continue with the tour as planned while I was having my surgery.

I decided that I would have immediate reconstruction after the mastectomy and that was done with implants. I had the choice to have a muscle taken from my back and moved into the breast area to avoid using implants, but to me it was far simpler to go down the implant route. At least that way I had only one area in my body to concentrate on healing. I'm sure some people would rather the feeling of a more natural breast made from your own tissue, but I wasn't bothered.

My mother was in Tenerife when I had the operation and she asked if I wanted her to come home, but I didn't. I wanted her to have some time for herself because she had been through so much and this was the first time that she had had a break from it all. My sister, Jo, came up from Galway and my friend, Martina, and my cousin, Robert, were all around to help and support me at that time. I wasn't sick, so it really wasn't a problem. I was just sore and I needed people to drive me here and there and lift things for me. Both Siobhán and Michael came home for weekends to visit me, but they both had to work so that was fine.

I was admitted into hospital the night before my surgery and, once again, I felt glad to be there because I knew that it was the final hurdle on my cancer journey. The surgery went well with no complications and I was so happy that it was all over. Although my new breasts didn't look the best at that stage, I was happy enough and I knew that they would improve over time. I was given plenty of painkillers so I was well able to cope with the discomfort.

After the fourth day in hospital, I decided to write a 'thank you' note and post it on Facebook to thank everyone who had sent letters and cards over the previous few months. Once again, the response was overwhelming, but when I started to get phone calls about newspaper and radio interviews, I wasn't sure how I should handle it. I know from previous interviews I have given, that your words can be misinterpreted and taken out of context, so I didn't want to do a newspaper interview. I also didn't want to be going onto every radio station to talk about my experience. I just wanted to keep my head down and get on with the job of healing my body.

Later on in the day, I was contacted by *The Late Late Show* to see if I would be interested in coming back to tell everyone how I was getting on. I thought that as I had started my journey with my head shave on the show, this would be a good way to round things up and at least I would be in control of what was being said and what people were hearing. I also wanted people to see that having a double mastectomy didn't mean that I would have to be locked away for weeks on end before I could bear to face the world again.

I did the show the day after I came out of hospital on the 21st of February and it wasn't a problem because I was on plenty of painkillers. As I was the first guest on that evening, I was home in my bed before the show finished that night. Ryan just asked how I was doing and what the surgery was like. It felt good to be there again where it had all started and to know that I was out the other side of it all. I had been completely bald when I finished the chemo in early December and by the time I was back on the show, I had a light covering of hair once again.

It was all over. I had done everything that I needed to do to to reduce the risk of my cancer returning.

When my father died, I thought that maybe he went so that he could keep an eye on me from up there and make sure nothing happened to me, but at the same time I thought, maybe he is gone because he is waiting for me. Who knows. I don't know that the timing of his death affected how I treated or felt about my illness. I don't think it did. That was just something separate that happened that I had to deal with. I am not the type to dwell on misfortunes any more. I did that for long enough after my marriage breakdown and I will never waste time in that way again. Things happen so I accept them and move on. Of course, that doesn't mean that I don't feel the loss of my father. I miss him very much and I still can't believe that he's gone, but I think of him in a happy way because I know that he is happy. Isn't that what we want for our loved ones? I think that mostly we feel sorry for ourselves after someone has died. Dad had a great life and he died the way he wanted to. There is so much to be grateful for and that's the way I cope with it.

I never, at any time during my journey, felt that cancer was going to get me. Even now I believe that I will never have to deal with it again. I hope I am right, but if it does return at any stage, I will deal with it in the same way. I suppose I feel confident that it won't come back because I caught it early and I did everything possible to increase my chances of it not returning. Of course, there are times when a little negative thought might creep in, but not for long. I don't allow myself down that road. In the meantime, I do not intend to spend my time worrying about whether it will return. Having said that, it is difficult not to worry when you have a new pain or a new lump or bump. That voice in your head always says, 'Hmm . . . I wonder if this is it, back again.' I will be very mindful of my body and watch out for changes, but I will not obsess over it. *Que sera, sera,* as the song says! Life is for living after all.

Chapter 10

THE FUTURE

So what does the future have in store for me? God only knows. On a personal note, I keep saying that I am such a lucky person because I am. I have lived a very full life – full enough for me anyway. I had a great childhood with lots of outdoor freedom and lots of friends. I lived in London for eight years and had a great time there. Then I moved to Scotland and lived there on and off for ten years and although there were tough times during that period, I have two beautiful children from that time and friends who will always be part of my life. I then moved to Tenerife, where I lived for two years and where my life changed completely. I was fortunate enough to spend quality time with my parents and I met my wonderful husband, Daniel. And now, life has come full circle with my move back to Ireland, which is something I had always wanted to do.

Healthwise, the future is anyone's guess. As I said just above, who knows what will happen in that regard. All I can do is to try to think positively and not to obsess about depression returning. Any time I do think, 'What if?' I soon realize what way my thinking is heading and I tell myself to let it go. Depression will always be part of my life, I believe. That's not to say that I will always be depressed. What I mean by that is that I will always have to be aware of it and watch out for it. It has been a few years now since I have had a bad bout of depression and I am grateful for that. I still take medication every day and as I tried on a few occasions to come off it without success, I am happy to continue on it for the rest of my life. It keeps me on an even keel, with no side effects. Not all people who suffer with depression can say the same. It can take a long time to find medication that works for you, but it's worth the effort to keep going until you find what suits you best.

I really can't explain how I ended up suffering from depression. When I was growing up, I was a very bubbly, chatty, enthusiastic and light-hearted child. I was always easy-going and never moody. My first episode happened when I was about twenty, although it was many years before

I actually went and did something about it. I just didn't recognize that depression was my problem. It's a form of mental illness and, as such, people are very fearful of it, which is crazy, really, because so many people suffer from it at one time or another. We all have our physical health and our mental health. At various times in our lives we have problems with our physical health, which need to be addressed: broken bones, skin conditions, eye problems, blood pressure, diabetes and so on. That's easy enough to deal with, in the sense that you can feel and touch and see your physical body. You know when something is not right with it. We don't have any problems going to our doctors to resolve physical problems. In any case, most physical problems *have* to be dealt with because they may incapacitate us if we ignore them. However, problems with our brains are seen very differently, which is a great pity. Why should it be any different? I think it's because the brain is such a complex organ and we know very little about it in comparison to our other organs. When we are ignorant about something, it can make us fearful.

The brain is like a computer and can do so many amazing things, but also, like a computer, it can go wrong. Depression incapacitates us in a very different way to physical problems: it is so difficult to describe to somebody how

you are when you're depressed. It is impossible to understand until you have been there yourself. It's a bit like trying
to describe what it's like to have a baby. Unless you have
experienced it, you cannot truly understand what it must
be like. Sometimes people think that it's like being really fed
up or 'down', but it's not like that at all. It is far more incap-
acitating. I can only describe it as like being down a very
deep, dark well or hole and you can see a little light at the
top; people are up there, looking down at you, but they can't
reach you and you can't reach them. You don't even want to
reach them. I can even have that feeling in a room full of
people. When I am in the grips of depression, I feel that
there is nothing in the world that can help me. I feel that I
am a burden to my family and to society. My thinking is
one of all-consuming blackness. It is the most awful feeling
in the world.

From my experience with both depression and cancer,
I can honestly say that depression was far worse to have to
deal with. Cancer is a 'thing'. You can attack it with drugs
and radiation and operations, but depression is very difficult to put your finger on or to try to treat. It's so hard even
to describe fully what your symptoms are! Also, when you
are physically sick, people are sympathetic towards you.
They offer to help you in any way they can. They ask about

you and worry about you because they have more of an understanding of what's happening to you, but when you're depressed, people don't know what to say or do. I can totally understand that. It is very hard to deal with a person with depression because there is very little you can do. I know that all I wanted was to know that someone was there if I needed them. I didn't want people trying to make me do things that might 'cheer me up' or trying to be overly cheery in the hope that I might 'snap out of it'. I just wanted to be left alone, but to know that I wasn't alone. There's a big difference between the two! I wanted someone to know that I was there and to try and reach out to me by maybe asking me to go for a walk or go to the pictures or something like that. I might not have wanted to go most of the time, but nevertheless I wanted to be asked because there is always the chance that one time I would feel up to it and that can be a turning point in the depression. As I have said, that is just how it is for me. Maybe other people would like to be handled very differently.

Thankfully, my bouts of depression these days are very few and far between. I'm very lucky that I have never been hospitalized for my depression. I try to stay on top of it by taking medication regularly and by being aware of my moods. I can usually tell if depression is coming, because I can almost see big black clouds heading towards me, so now I try to do something before they take hold. Sometimes that doesn't work and I know that I just have to ride out the storm and know that it will end. I tell myself that constantly when I'm depressed. 'This, too, will end.' It is a struggle to believe that because, when you have been there before, you are always afraid that this time it may not go away, but it always has in my case and that's what I need to remind myself at those low points. There is no quick fix with mental-health issues. You just have to be aware of your moods and your behaviour and to keep yourself in check.

Stress, in my opinion, is one of the worst causes of depression. I fight stress by being in nature as much as I can. Daniel and I have an old cottage on the island of Owey, and being there is a great stress reliever. There is no electricity or running water, there are no cars and no roads. Life was physically very tough indeed for the people that lived there throughout the year. It was a hard slog to just get by and provide for your family. When I go out there I notice how relaxed I become. There are no distractions. No television or computers. All the normal things that we take for granted are gone, so it takes longer to do everything. You have to boil a kettle to wash yourself. Everything is washed by hand, but I notice that there is no stress. When you go to bed at night you are exhausted just from the day's work, but you are never stressed. I think that our modern lifestyle has lead to this new illness we know as stress and, ironically, we have brought it upon ourselves. In our quest to have an easier lifestyle, we have created the monster that is more commonly known as 'stress'. Also, technology has progressed at such an incredible rate that we can hardly keep up with it. In the past, things were much slower in every respect. Nowadays things are instant. Like email. No more having to wait for the post: technology has given us the power to be able to do things straightaway and, of course, we have embraced that, but the downside is that we can never get away from it now. Before mobile phones, you didn't just call someone and expect to get them. You had to wait if they were not there for the day and you accepted that. Now, if I call Daniel or Siobhán and I don't get them after a couple of calls, I'm annoyed and impatient. 'What's the point in you having a mobile phone if you don't answer it?' is my usual gripe.

I'm not saying that it's a bad thing. It's just the way it is, but we have to be aware of it and not let it overcome us. We need to stay in touch with the simple things in life and to appreciate them more. We need to get out and communicate with other human beings more and not be constantly living in a 'cyber' world, which is very easy to do. You don't have to leave your settee and yet you can shop and talk to people from every corner of the earth and you can find out about absolutely everything you ever wanted to know. It's absolutely fantastic really, but we mustn't lose sight of the important things in life, like community. We have all that information at our fingertips, yet we are alone in a room. We think that we have loads of friends, but it's not 'real'. No wonder people get depressed. My advice is to look forward and to embrace the new, but to cherish the values of the past and to try and integrate the two whenever we can.

Of course, I understand that there are other reasons why people might be depressed. In my case, I have clinical depression, which is caused by an imbalance of hormones in my brain. Sometimes an event can trigger it, but more often than not, there is no reason at all why this big black cloud decides to descend upon me. I suppose if I am stressed out or doing too much it is more likely to happen, so I try to have as much quiet time in my life as I can.

I wish that society in general would be more accepting of mental-health issues. My goal is to do my bit to help in that regard. The more we speak about these issues, the more 'normal' they will become. Huge research also needs to be done in the medical and psychiatric fields to better under-stand this problem and to understand our brains. I don't think that psychiatric medicine is a particularly 'stylish' or 'trendy' field to be in, but perhaps that's changing as stress and depression become more and more a part of our lives.

Having experienced depression at first hand and having come through a marriage breakdown and cancer, I wanted to use what I had learned to help other people in similar situations. As I said in my introduction, I have given talks about my experience in the past and they have been warmly received. I have always been told that I articulate my experi-ence very well and that people seem to relate to me. As I have no problem speaking to people, I think that maybe this is my role in life. I really enjoy it. It has come about quite by accident, but it's changed my life for the better. Also, I have been working with a group in Donegal, which forms part of the Health Service Executive, for a couple of years now and we are in the process of setting up a charity, which we have called Donegal Mind Wellness or 'DMW' for short. We aim to raise funds that can be used to reach out to people who are stressed or depressed or feel they can't cope. Donegal is such a remote area of Ireland and it has been hit by so many tragedies and bad unemployment over the years. There are a few people involved in the charity, but I suppose the main driving force behind it would be Anne Sheridan, Mental Health Promotion/Suicide Resource Officer for the HSE in the north-west of Ireland. All the people giving the courses are volunteers and I am extremely grateful to them and proud of them for what they are giving back to others. We could not do this without them. We have already started a six-week course in stress management that anyone can attend, free of charge, to give them the tools to help them to cope better in times of stress. It's been hugely successful so far.

Stress can and usually does include nervousness, anxiety, tension, distress, grief, strain, pressure, trauma and difficulty coping, which can all led to depression. This is why we need to learn ways of handling our stress. We will never eliminate it altogether, but we can control it with the right tools. I am very excited about it and I encourage anyone in the area to look out for it and if you don't think it's something you could benefit from, then maybe you know someone else who might. Personally, I think we can all benefit from it and I have taken the course myself, so I know what I'm talking about.

Once, when I had a one-to-one session with Jack Black, the founder of MindStore, he asked me this question: 'If you were on your death bed and God came to you and granted you an extra ten years onto your life, what would you do with it?' I thought long and hard and I realized that there really wasn't anything else I needed to do in life. I have travelled a lot, I have lived in different countries, I have a wonderful partner and two beautiful children, I have released two albums and now I am writing a book! I told him that I would be happy to continue as I was and just have more of the same in my life. He thought it was an unusual answer because, he told me, most people reel off a list of things that they would like to do if they get a second chance, if they get those extra ten years. The point of that exercise is to show people that whatever it is you want to do in your life, you should do it now, or at least plan for it now. Don't wait until the last day, when it'll be too late.

It really did make me think about my life and I realized that I was very happy. I *am* very happy! Sure, I have my ups and downs but, in a general sense, I am very content. I am such a lucky person. The last fourteen years of my life, since I met Daniel, have been very happy, peaceful years. I have been blessed with so much in my life. In particular, it has also been wonderful to be reintroduced to music since meeting Daniel. I had one party-piece song that I used to sing called 'Walkin' After Midnight' by Patsy Cline and Daniel surprised me one day by asking me to come on stage and sing it. At the time I was in his dressing room sewing a pair of trousers with my slippers on. So off I went on stage, in my slippers and all, and sang the song. That was in Dallas, Texas, in front of an audience of 2,000 people and I'll never forget it.

Daniel is very cool and calm on stage. Nothing seems to faze him. So he had no problem asking me to join him on the stage when I was totally unprepared, but it didn't bother me really. It was all a bit of fun. Nobody was expecting me to be any good anyway. Unfortunately, I have a genuine problem as far as performing is concerned. I cannot retain the words of songs after I have learned them. If I don't sing something for a few weeks, it's gone from my memory. Daniel could sing a song that he only heard on the radio once or twice! Or something that he learned twenty years ago. On top of that, the nerves don't help either, so it can make for a very unpleasant experience. If I have the words written down in front of me, I'm happy as Larry.

Before we were married I went to a recording studio with Daniel for the first time. I couldn't take it all in. I loved being there and watching how everything worked. The guys, engineer Daire Winston and producer John Ryan, knew that I could sing a bit, so when Daniel finished what he was recording they asked me if I wanted to go into the recording room and sing something. I was delighted and apprehensive at the same time. I might love singing, but I'd never heard myself, so I might have been very disappointed. I sang 'Crazy', another song by Patsy Cline, and that was it. John said that they would put some music to it and let me hear it sometime. The recording studio is very busy so I really didn't expect to hear anything and I just thought they were humouring me.

Months passed and I had forgotten all about that day, but on our wedding day Daire came up to me and handed me a gift. To my absolute delight, it was a CD with me singing 'Crazy' on it. That was the first time that I had really heard my own voice and it wasn't bad. I think that the more you sing, the better your voice becomes. You are using muscles, so the more exercise they get, the better for your voice. If I had had a career in singing years ago, I might have been a pretty good singer, if I say so myself!

However, what music I listen to and what suits my voice are two different things. My voice suits country and a bit of the blues, but that's not what I would listen to. My taste in music is very eclectic, with artists such as Bob Marley, Barbara Streisand, The Fureys, Dolores Keane, The Eagles, Mary and Frances Black, Imelda May and lots more being top of my list. In fact, anything that I consider soulful. All very varied, depending on the mood I'm in. Daniel sings a song called 'Red Is The Rose', a traditional Irish song and I have to say that it's one of the most soulful, beautiful songs that I have ever heard him singing. When I listen to it, it has such a calming effect on me. I don't think you can say that because you don't like something musically that it's no good. It may not be to *your* taste, but that doesn't mean it's no good. If it makes *you* feel good then it's good for you and that's all that matters.

You really never know what the future holds for you because I would never in my wildest dreams have believed that I would get the opportunity to record a duet with Sir Cliff Richard, but I did. We were away on a cruise together with a group of friends and I was telling them that I was recording an album. One of them said, 'Why don't you two record a duet?' pointing to Cliff and me. We started talking about it and Cliff suggested a song, 'He Knows, She Knows'. We went to a studio and recorded it and I was so impressed with Cliff because he was so enthusiastic and really wanted it to be as good as it could be. It didn't matter that I wasn't a huge recording artist. So, thank you for that, Cliff! I'm pretty sure that I won't record again, although they do say never say never. I just feel that I have other things that I am more interested in doing, but who knows. That's all in the future.

I have experienced so much in my life that I really don't have any great 'bucket list' of things that I would like to do. There are a few things and I have included them in my goals. As I mentioned, I have set up 'Donegal Mind Wellness' to help people with stress and depression in Donegal. I really want to travel to Venice and Amsterdam sometime soon, but one of my biggest desires in life is that my children will be happy. I suppose that's the wish of any parent. I always thought that once I had reared my children, I would wave them goodbye as they sailed into the sunset to live their lives, only coming back now and then for family dinners or breaks. How naïve that was! I realize now that I will never stop worrying about my kids. They will always be my babies, even though they are now adults. If they are alone, I worry that they are lonely and that they might not meet someone. Then, when they do meet some-one, I worry that it won't work out and that they might get hurt. It's never-ending, but I suppose that's what a mother's job is. I can't wait to have grandchildren and that's assum-ing that I will, which may not be the case. Who knows? But I think I will be a far better grandmother than I was a mother. I will have more time to concentrate on my grandchildren than I did my own children, even though at the time, I did my very best. I never wanted anything from my children, but to be the best they can be at whatever it is they want to do. To be happy and to be able to support themselves in life. That's when I feel I will have done my job as a mother. Our role is to support them in whatever it is that they want to do, to be there for them when things go wrong and to teach them to be decent human beings.

There is nothing else that I want from life, but hopefully to stay healthy and to continue my journey with Daniel, Siobhán, Michael and my family and friends. I am very happy with the simple things in life now and I really don't need much to survive. I enjoy nature and the beauty of it; I love being outdoors in the fresh air; but I don't mind wrapping up against the cold, even though I do hate the constant grey drizzle that we get during the winter in Ireland. I love open fires and feeling cosy on a cold winter's night. I am not a great person for the sun, but I love a blue sky. What more do I need?